50 Myths About Diets & Weight Loss

Debunking Common Misconceptions for a Healthier, Smarter Approach to Weight Management

The Insight Collective

Published by *Insightful Press.*

"50 Myths About..." Series
Book #2: Diets & Weight Loss

ISBN: 9798332628542

First Edition

Contents

Access Additional Resources Online

For your convenience, all the external links referenced in this book and the comprehensive bibliography are available online. Visit our dedicated website to explore further and deepen your understanding of the fascinating world of diets.

Scan the QR codes below to access:

External Links:

Comprehensive Bibliography:

Alternatively, you can visit:

External Links:

https://50mythsabout.blogspot.com/2024/07/50-myths-about-diets-weight-loss.html

Comprehensive Bibliography:

https://50mythsabout.blogspot.com/2024/07/50-myths-about-diets-weight-loss_8.html

Enhance your reading experience and discover more about the myths and realities of architecture.

"The greatest wealth is health."

— Virgil

Introduction:
Debunking Diet and Weight Loss Myths

In a world overflowing with diet trends, weight loss fads, and nutritional advice, it's easy to feel overwhelmed and confused about what truly works. From celebrity endorsements to miracle supplements, the diet industry bombards us with promises of quick fixes and easy solutions. But how much of what we hear is actually true?

This book is your guide to cutting through the noise and finding evidence-based information that will empower you to make informed decisions about your health and wellness.

Over the years, many myths have taken root in the collective consciousness, leading to widespread misconceptions about dieting and weight loss. These myths can derail your progress, foster unhealthy habits, and leave you feeling frustrated and disillusioned. Our goal is to set the record straight by exploring and debunking 50 of the most pervasive myths in the diet and weight loss world.

We'll delve into topics like carbs, fats, meal timing, exercise, and more, providing clear explanations and practical advice along the way. Whether you're just starting your weight loss journey or looking to refine your approach, this book offers valuable insights to help you achieve sustainable, long-term success.

Remember, achieving and maintaining a healthy weight isn't about following the latest trends or adhering to rigid rules—it's about understanding your body's needs, making mindful choices, and cultivating a balanced lifestyle. Let's embark on this journey together and uncover the truths that will lead you to a healthier, happier you.

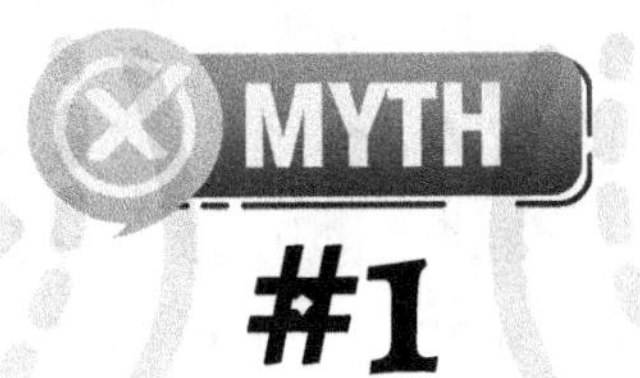

Carbs are bad for weight loss

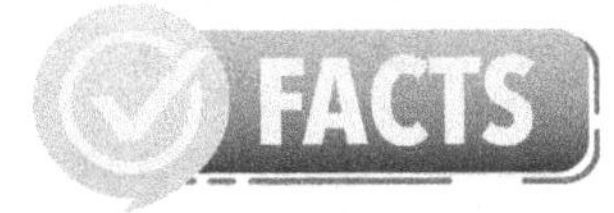

Not all carbs are created equal. Complex carbs provide sustained energy.

The notion that carbohydrates are inherently bad for weight loss is a common myth that oversimplifies the complex nature of carbs. The truth is, not all carbs are created equal, and understanding the differences between them can significantly impact your weight management and overall health.

Carbohydrates can be broadly categorized into simple and complex carbs. Simple carbs, such as those found in sugary snacks and refined grains, are quickly digested, leading to rapid spikes in blood sugar and subsequent energy crashes. In contrast, complex carbs, which are found in whole grains, legumes, vegetables, and fruits, are digested more slowly, providing a steady release of energy. This gradual energy release helps maintain stable blood sugar levels and prevents the fatigue often associated with high-sugar diets.

In terms of weight management, complex carbs are typically more filling and satisfying due to their higher fiber content. Fiber adds bulk to your meals, promoting a feeling of fullness and reducing the likelihood of overeating. Additionally, fiber aids in digestion, supports a healthy gut microbiome, and helps regulate blood sugar levels, all of which are beneficial for weight control and overall health.

Moreover, the quality of carbohydrates consumed plays a crucial role. Diets rich in minimally processed carbs, such as whole grains, fruits, and legumes, are associated with numerous health benefits, including improved heart health, better blood sugar control, and enhanced digestion. These foods are packed with essential nutrients like vitamins, minerals, and antioxidants, which support various bodily functions and contribute to long-term well-being.

It's also a misconception that carbs should be avoided entirely if you have diabetes or that consuming them at night leads to weight gain. Instead, focusing on the type of carbs and their timing can help manage blood sugar levels and support weight loss efforts without eliminating this vital macronutrient from your diet.

In conclusion, while it's essential to limit intake of refined carbs and sugary foods, incorporating complex carbs into your diet can provide sustained energy, improve satiety, and support overall health. Choosing high-quality, fiber-rich carbs is key to achieving and maintaining a healthy weight and lifestyle.

External links:

Eat This Not That — 15 Myths About Carbohydrates You Should Stop Believing

https://www.eatthis.com/carbohydrates-myths/

Bodybuilding Wizard — Unmasking the Myths: Debunking Common Misconceptions about Carbohydrates

https://bodybuilding-wizard.com/myths-misconceptions-about-carbohydrates-debunked/

Precision Nutrition — All About Carbs: Facts & Myths

https://www.precisionnutrition.com/all-about-carbohydrates

Cleveland Clinic — Good vs. Bad Carbs: What Should You Eat?

https://health.clevelandclinic.org/good-carb-bad-carb-dont-buy-into-4-myths

MyAuthentikSpoon — Myth vs. Reality: Are carbs bad for you?

https://myauthentikspoon.com/myth-vs-reality-are-carbs-bad-for-you/

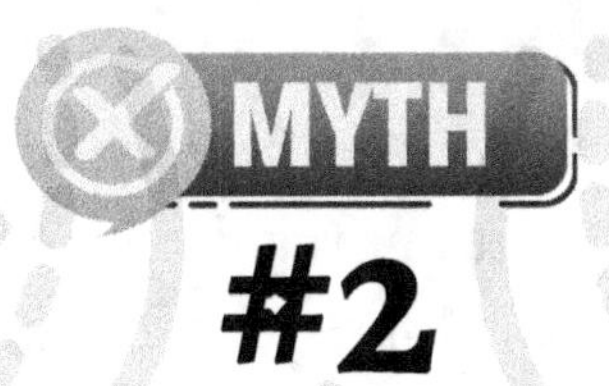

Skipping meals helps you lose weight

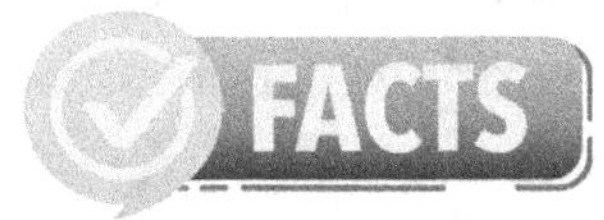

Skipping meals can slow down your metabolism and lead to overeating later.

The idea that skipping meals helps with weight loss is a widespread myth. In reality, skipping meals can have counterproductive effects, including slowing down your metabolism and leading to overeating later in the day.

When you skip meals, your body goes into a conservation mode, slowing down your metabolism to conserve energy. This adaptive response is designed to protect the body during times of food scarcity, but it can make weight loss more difficult by reducing the number of calories your body burns at rest.

Moreover, skipping meals often leads to intense hunger, which can cause you to overeat at subsequent meals. This pattern of eating can result in consuming more calories than if you had eaten regular, balanced meals throughout the day. Research shows that people who skip meals are more likely to make poor food choices and consume larger portions when they finally eat, often choosing high-calorie, low-nutrient foods.

Regular meals help maintain stable blood sugar levels, which is crucial for controlling hunger and energy levels. Eating balanced meals that include a mix of proteins, fats, and complex carbohydrates can help you feel fuller longer, reducing the temptation to snack on unhealthy foods.

Additionally, skipping meals can negatively impact your mood and cognitive function. Low blood sugar levels from not eating can lead to irritability, fatigue, and difficulty concentrating, making it harder to stick to healthy eating and exercise habits.

For sustainable weight loss, it's better to focus on portion control and making healthy food choices rather than skipping meals. Eating regular, well-balanced meals supports a higher metabolism and helps prevent the overeating that often follows periods of food deprivation.

In summary, while it might seem like an easy way to cut calories, skipping meals can backfire, making weight loss harder and potentially leading to weight gain in the long run. Instead, aim for balanced meals and snacks throughout the day to support a healthy metabolism and overall well-being.

⤴ External links:

Anytime Fitness — 10 Common Weight-Loss Myths, Busted
https://www.anytimefitness.com/ccc/ask-a-coach/common-weight-loss-myths-busted/

Hindustan Times — From skipping meals to crash diets: Debunking the top weight loss myths
https://www.hindustantimes.com/lifestyle/health/from-skipping-meals-to-crash-diets-debunking-the-top-weight-loss-myths-101674018943636.html

SMW Blog — Blog - 10 Common Myths About Weight Loss Debunked
https://sportsmedicineweekly.com/blog/10-common-myths-about-weight-loss-debunked/

stack — Food Myths Busted: Skipping Meals Helps You Lose Weight
https://www.stack.com/a/skipping-meals/

Nutritionist Resource — Weight-loss nutrition myths debunked
https://www.nutritionist-resource.org.uk/memberarticles/weight-loss-nutrition-myths-debunked

Piedmont HealthCare — What Happens to the Body When You Skip Meals?
https://www.piedmont.org/living-real-change/what-happens-to-the-body-when-you-skip-meals

Have A Plant — About The Buzz: Skipping Meals Will Help With Weight Loss
https://fruitsandveggies.org/stories/about-the-buzz-skipping-meals-will-help-with-weight-loss/

WeightMatters — Skipping meals for weight loss | Does it work?
https://weightmatters.ie/skipping-meals-for-weight-loss/

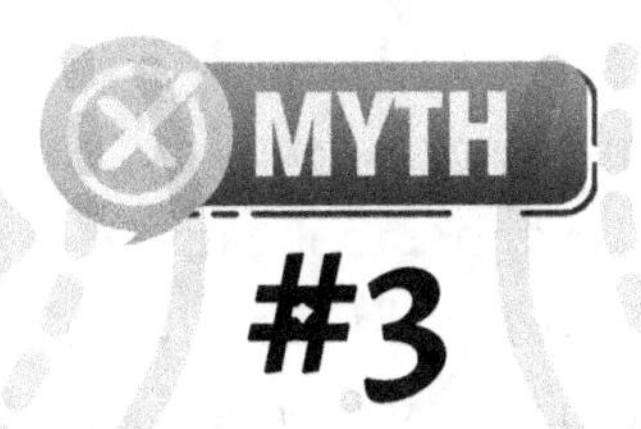

All calories are equal

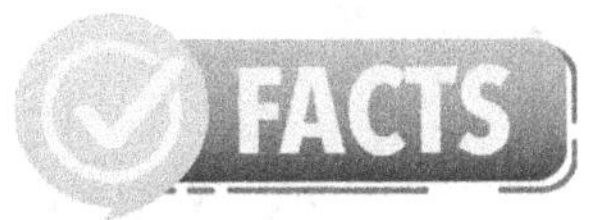

The source of calories matters. 200 calories of vegetables are not the same as 200 calories of candy.

The notion that all calories are equal is a myth. While the calorie is a unit of energy, the source of those calories plays a crucial role in how they affect your body. Consuming 200 calories from vegetables versus 200 calories from candy leads to vastly different physiological responses.

Vegetables are packed with fiber, vitamins, and minerals, which support digestion, enhance satiety, and promote overall health. On the other hand, candy is high in simple sugars, which cause rapid spikes in blood sugar and insulin levels, leading to increased hunger and potential overeating later.

The thermic effect of food (TEF), which is the energy expenditure required for digestion, varies between macronutrients. Protein has a higher TEF compared to fats and carbohydrates, meaning the body burns more calories processing protein. This contributes to why calories from different sources can have different impacts on metabolism and weight management (Hindustan Times).

Furthermore, the glycemic index (GI) is a measure of how quickly foods raise blood sugar levels. Foods high on the GI, such as candy, lead to rapid glucose spikes and subsequent crashes, while low-GI foods, like most vegetables, provide a slower, more sustained release of energy. Diets high in low-GI foods are associated with better weight management and metabolic health.

Processed foods, often high in simple sugars and refined carbs, can lead to a slower metabolism and increased risk of weight gain and metabolic diseases. Conversely, whole foods, which are nutrient-dense and low in the glycemic index, help maintain stable blood sugar levels, support metabolism, and promote overall health.

In conclusion, while a calorie is a calorie in terms of energy content, the source of those calories significantly affects your health. Prioritizing nutrient-dense, whole foods over processed, high-sugar foods is crucial for effective weight management and overall well-being.

External links:

livescience.com — When Dieting, Not All Calories Are Created Equal
https://www.livescience.com/21192-calories-not-equal-best-diets.html

Hindustan Times — From skipping meals to crash diets: Debunking the top weight loss myths
https://www.hindustantimes.com/lifestyle/health/from-skipping-meals-to-crash-diets-debunking-the-top-weight-loss-myths-101674018943636.html

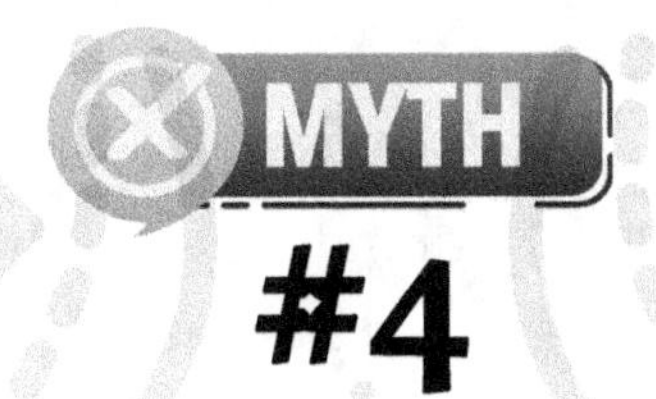

Fat makes you fat

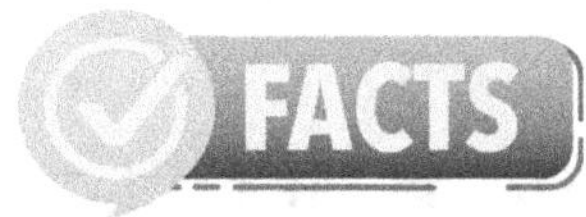

Healthy fats, like those found in avocados and nuts, are essential for a balanced diet.

The myth that fat makes you fat has been debunked by numerous studies and health experts. While it's true that all fats are calorie-dense, not all fats are created equal. Healthy fats, such as those found in avocados, nuts, and olive oil, are essential for a balanced diet and overall health.

Healthy fats, including monounsaturated and polyunsaturated fats, play crucial roles in the body. They are vital for building cell membranes, supporting nerve function, and helping the body absorb fat-soluble vitamins like A, D, E, and K. For instance, omega-3 fatty acids found in fatty fish, nuts, and seeds are particularly beneficial for heart and brain health.

Consuming healthy fats can actually aid in weight management. These fats help you feel fuller longer, which can prevent overeating and snacking on unhealthy foods. Additionally, they have been shown to improve metabolic health and reduce the risk of chronic diseases such as heart disease and diabetes.

In contrast, unhealthy fats, such as trans fats and excessive saturated fats, can contribute to weight gain and health issues. Trans fats, often found in processed foods, are particularly harmful and have been linked to increased risks of heart disease and inflammation. The FDA has banned artificial trans fats due to their adverse health effects.

It's important to distinguish between different types of fats and incorporate healthy fats into your diet while limiting unhealthy ones. By doing so, you can support your overall health, maintain a balanced diet, and effectively manage your weight.

⧉ **External links:**

Fact / Myth — Fat Makes You Fat - Fact or Myth?
https://factmyth.com/factoids/fat-makes-you-fat/

HealthBehavSci — Debunking 10 Common Nutrition Myths - Faculty of Health and Behavioural Sciences - University of Queensland
https://habs.uq.edu.au/blog/2023/10/debunking-10-common-nutrition-myths

The Healthy — Myths About Fat You Need to Stop Believing
https://www.thehealthy.com/weight-loss/myths-about-fat/

Bodybuilding — 10 Nutrition Myths Debunked
https://www.bodybuilding.com/content/10-nutrition-myths-debunked.html

Cleveland Clinic — Do Fats Make You Fat?
https://health.clevelandclinic.org/all-about-fats-why-you-need-them-in-your-diet

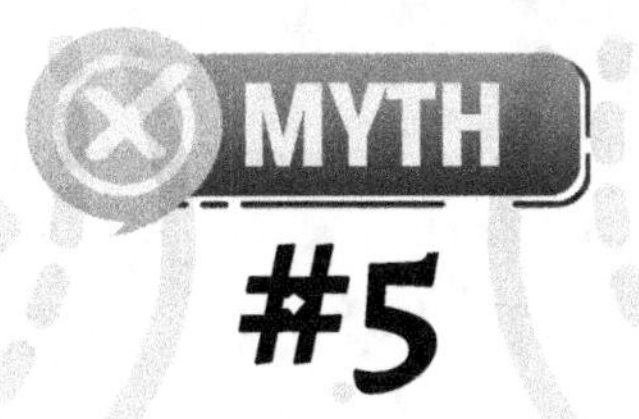

You need to eat special diet foods to lose weight

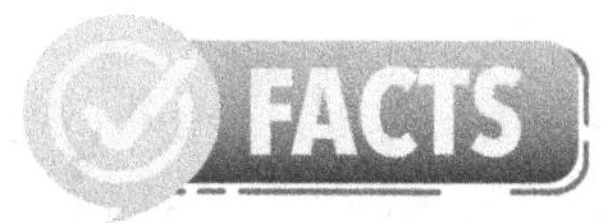

Whole, unprocessed foods are often the best choice for weight loss.

The belief that special diet foods are necessary for weight loss is a myth. In reality, whole, unprocessed foods are often the best choice for achieving and maintaining a healthy weight.

Whole foods, such as fruits, vegetables, whole grains, lean proteins, and healthy fats, provide essential nutrients that support overall health and weight management. These foods are rich in fiber, which aids in digestion and helps you feel full longer, reducing the likelihood of overeating. For example, a study highlighted by Everyday Health found that participants who followed a whole-foods, plant-based diet for six months lost about 10 pounds, while a control group lost less than a pound. This weight loss was maintained over a year, showcasing the effectiveness of whole foods in weight management.

Processed diet foods, on the other hand, often contain added sugars, unhealthy fats, and artificial ingredients. These components can contribute to weight gain and other health issues. For instance, many gluten-free processed foods, while essential for those with celiac disease, can be higher in calories and lower in fiber than their whole food counterparts, potentially leading to weight gain over time.

Eating whole foods also helps regulate blood sugar levels, supports a healthy gut microbiome, and provides a steady source of energy. This contrasts with processed foods, which can cause spikes and crashes in blood sugar, leading to increased hunger and cravings.

Incorporating a variety of whole foods into your diet doesn't just help with weight loss; it also promotes long-term health by providing a broad spectrum of nutrients necessary for bodily functions. For example, including sources of healthy fats like avocados and nuts can support heart health and improve satiety.

In summary, focusing on whole, unprocessed foods is a more effective and sustainable approach to weight loss compared to relying on special diet foods. This approach not only helps in shedding pounds but also enhances overall health and well-being.

External links:

Cleveland Clinic — 6 Worst Myths You've Ever Heard About Weight Loss
https://health.clevelandclinic.org/6-worst-myths-youve-ever-heard-about-weight-loss

EverydayHealth.com — What Is a Whole-Foods Diet? Benefits, Risks, Food List, and More
https://www.everydayhealth.com/diet-nutrition/whole-foods-diet/

nhs.uk — Healthy eating when trying to lose weight - Better Health
https://www.nhs.uk/better-health/lose-weight/healthy-eating-when-trying-to-lose-weight/

Livestrong.com — The Whole Foods Weight Loss Eating Plan
https://www.livestrong.com/article/294064-the-whole-foods-weight-loss-eating-plan/

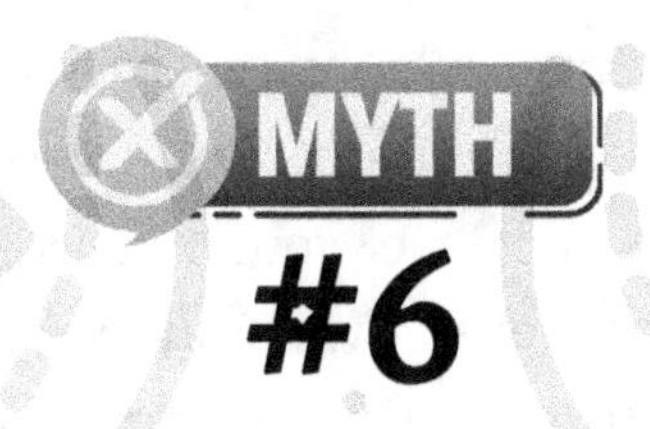

Exercise alone is enough for weight loss

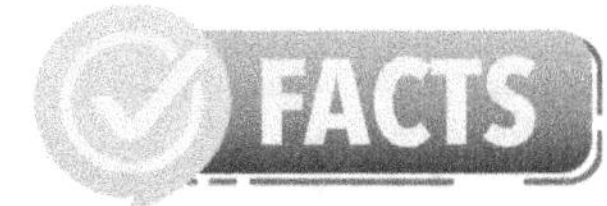

Exercise is important, but diet plays a crucial role in weight loss.

The belief that exercise alone is sufficient for weight loss is a common myth. While exercise is an important component of a healthy lifestyle and offers numerous benefits, including improving cardiovascular health, building muscle, and enhancing mental well-being, it is not the sole factor in weight loss. Diet plays a crucial role in achieving and maintaining a healthy weight.

Research has consistently shown that creating a calorie deficit—burning more calories than you consume—is essential for weight loss. This can be achieved through a combination of diet and exercise. For instance, even though exercise burns calories, the amount burned during typical exercise sessions is often less significant compared to the calories consumed through diet. Therefore, focusing solely on exercise without addressing dietary habits may not lead to substantial weight loss.

Studies have demonstrated that individuals who combine a healthy diet with regular exercise are more successful in losing weight and keeping it off than those who rely on exercise alone. A balanced diet rich in whole, unprocessed foods like fruits, vegetables, whole grains, lean proteins, and healthy fats supports weight loss by providing essential nutrients and promoting satiety, which helps prevent overeating.

Furthermore, the type of exercise matters. While cardiovascular exercises like running and cycling are effective for burning calories, strength training is also crucial as it builds muscle mass, which can increase your resting metabolic rate. This means you burn more calories even when at rest. Incorporating both cardio and strength training into your fitness routine, along with a nutritious diet, is the most effective strategy for weight loss.

In conclusion, while exercise is vital for overall health and supports weight management, it must be combined with a healthy diet to achieve and maintain weight loss. A holistic approach that includes balanced nutrition, regular physical activity, and other healthy lifestyle choices is key to effective and sustainable weight loss.

External links:

NutritionFacts.org — The Exercise "Myth" for Weight Loss
https://nutritionfacts.org/video/the-exercise-myth-for-weight-loss/

Lean Body Goals — The Role of Exercise in Weight Management: Myth vs. Reality
https://leanbodygoals.com/the-role-of-exercise-in-weight-management-myth-vs-reality/

Cleveland Clinic — Weight Loss: Can You Do It With Exercise Alone?
https://health.clevelandclinic.org/weight-loss-can-you-do-it-with-exercise-alone

PBMC Health — Is Exercise Alone Enough for Weight Loss?
https://www.pbmchealth.org/news-events/blog/exercise-alone-enough-weight-loss

ScienceDaily — Exercise alone does not help in losing weight
https://www.sciencedaily.com/releases/2015/08/150817142140.htm

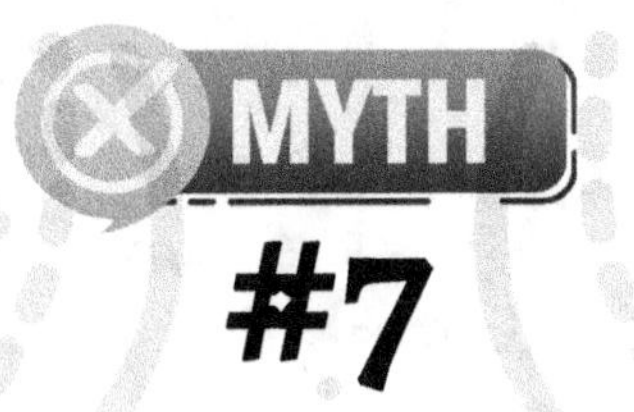

Eating after 8 PM or late at night causes weight gain

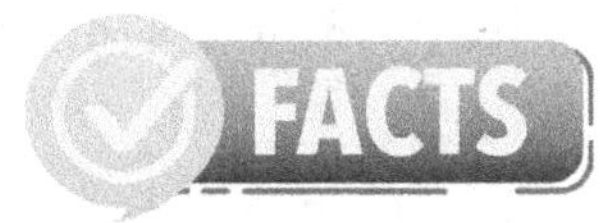

The timing of eating has less impact than the total daily intake of calories.

The idea that eating after 8 PM or late at night inherently causes weight gain is a myth. The more crucial factor in weight management is the total daily intake of calories rather than the timing of meals.

Research has shown that while late-night eating can be associated with weight gain, it is not the time itself but the potential for increased calorie consumption and poorer food choices that contribute to this effect. For instance, people who eat late at night might be more inclined to consume high-calorie, nutrient-poor snacks like chips or sweets, which can lead to an excess calorie intake.

Moreover, late-night eating can disrupt the body's natural circadian rhythms, which regulate hormones related to hunger and metabolism. Studies indicate that eating later in the evening can alter the levels of hunger-regulating hormones, such as leptin and ghrelin, leading to increased appetite and reduced satiety. This hormonal imbalance can make it easier to overeat, thereby promoting weight gain over time.

Another aspect to consider is the body's metabolic response to late eating. Some studies have found that consuming meals late at night can slow down the rate at which calories are burned, further contributing to weight gain. For example, a study by researchers at Harvard found that late eating decreased the number of calories burned the following day and promoted fat storage at the molecular level.

However, it is essential to emphasize that the overall daily caloric intake is the primary factor in weight management. If the total calories consumed in a day are within the body's energy needs, the timing of meals has less impact on weight gain. Therefore, focusing on balanced, nutritious meals throughout the day and maintaining an overall caloric deficit is more effective for weight loss than simply avoiding late-night eating.

In conclusion, while late-night eating can contribute to weight gain due to hormonal disruptions and poor food choices, it is the total daily calorie intake that ultimately determines weight management. Emphasizing a balanced diet and mindful eating habits throughout the day is key to effective weight control.

External links:

Harvard Gazette — Study looks at why late-night eating increases obesity risk
https://news.harvard.edu/gazette/story/2022/10/study-looks-at-why-late-night-eating-increases-obesity-risk/

Med Xpress — Late night eating may cause greater weight gain: New research points to why
https://medicalxpress.com/news/2022-10-late-night-greater-weight-gain.html

Penn Medicine — Timing Meals Later at Night Can Cause Weight Gain and Impair Fat Metabolism
https://www.pennmedicine.org/news/news-releases/2017/june/timing-meals-later-at-night-can-cause-weight-gain-and-impair-fat-metabolism

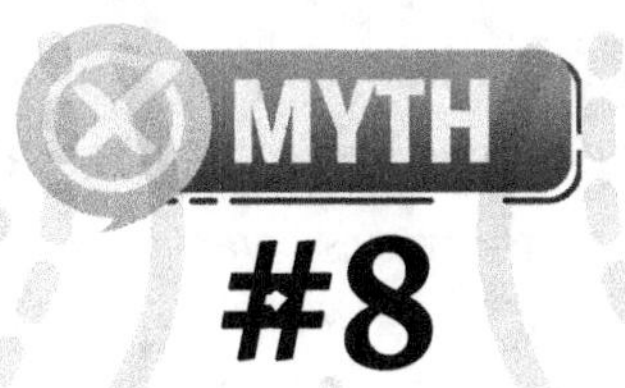

Detox diets and juicing are necessary for weight loss

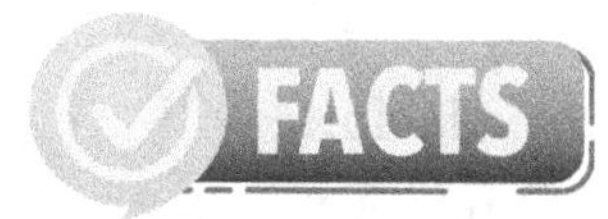

Your body naturally detoxifies itself. Juicing and detox diets are not necessary.

The belief that detox diets and juicing are necessary for weight loss is a widespread myth. In reality, your body is fully equipped to detoxify itself naturally, and these diets are not required for effective weight management.

The body's primary detoxification systems involve the liver, kidneys, and gastrointestinal (GI) tract. These organs work continuously to eliminate toxins and waste products from the body without the need for special diets or cleanses. The liver, for instance, processes toxins and converts them into substances that can be safely excreted. Similarly, the kidneys filter blood to remove waste products through urine, and the GI tract eliminates solid waste.

Detox diets and juice cleanses often promise quick weight loss, but these effects are usually temporary and primarily due to a significant reduction in calorie intake and loss of water weight. Such diets can lead to muscle loss, nutrient deficiencies, and other health issues if followed for extended periods. Once normal eating patterns resume, the lost weight is often quickly regained.

Moreover, juice cleanses can lack essential nutrients like protein and fiber, leading to potential side effects such as low energy, headaches, and digestive issues like constipation. They may also disrupt blood sugar levels, causing irritability and fatigue.

Long-term, sustainable weight loss and overall health are best supported by maintaining a balanced diet rich in whole, unprocessed foods, regular physical activity, and proper hydration. Foods such as fruits, vegetables, whole grains, lean proteins, and healthy fats provide the necessary nutrients to support your body's natural detoxification processes and overall health.

In conclusion, while detox diets and juicing may offer short-term weight loss, they are not effective or necessary for long-term health. Your body is naturally equipped to detoxify itself, and the best approach to weight loss involves a balanced diet and healthy lifestyle choices.

↗ **External links:**

MD Anderson Cancer Center — Should you detox your body? 4 myths about detoxing
https://www.mdanderson.org/cancerwise/the-facts-behind-4-detox-myths-should-you-detox-your-body.hoo-159385890.html

Ask The Scientists — Fact or Fiction: Making Sense of Detox Myths
https://askthescientists.com/detox-myths/

NCCIH — "Detoxes" and "Cleanses": What You Need To Know
https://www.nccih.nih.gov/health/detoxes-and-cleanses-what-you-need-to-know

livescience.com — 4 Myths About Juice Cleansing
https://www.livescience.com/48767-juice-cleanse-myths.html

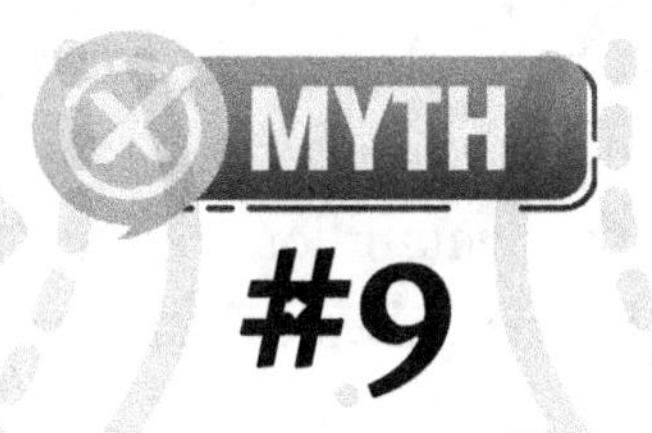

Drinking lots of water leads to weight loss

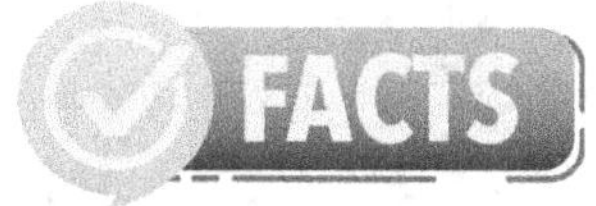

Drinking water is important for health, but it won't cause significant weight loss alone.

The belief that drinking lots of water directly leads to weight loss is a common myth. While staying hydrated is crucial for overall health, it does not cause significant weight loss by itself.

Water plays several essential roles in the body, including maintaining hydration, aiding digestion, and regulating body temperature. Drinking water can help you feel full, which might reduce your overall calorie intake if consumed before meals. For example, some studies suggest that drinking water before meals can slightly reduce appetite and help with weight management in conjunction with a healthy diet and exercise.

However, the effect of water on metabolism and calorie burning is minimal. Although there is evidence that drinking water can temporarily boost metabolism, the impact is small and not sufficient to cause significant weight loss on its own. A study found that drinking 500 ml of water increased resting energy expenditure by about 24 percent for only an hour, which translates to a very modest calorie burn.

Additionally, while water can aid in the body's natural detoxification processes through the kidneys and urinary tract, it does not melt away fat or result in long-term weight loss. Effective and sustainable weight loss requires a combination of factors, including a balanced diet, regular physical activity, and lifestyle changes.

In summary, while drinking water is vital for health and can support weight loss efforts as part of a comprehensive approach, it is not a standalone solution for significant weight loss. Ensuring proper hydration is beneficial, but focusing on a well-rounded diet and consistent exercise regimen is essential for achieving and maintaining a healthy weight.

External links:

The Hub — Yes, drinking more water may help you lose weight
https://hub.jhu.edu/at-work/2020/01/15/focus-on-wellness-drinking-more-water/

ScienceDaily — Debunking water myths: Weight loss, calorie burn and more
https://www.sciencedaily.com/releases/2014/03/140312132315.htm

EverydayHealth.com — Can You Lose Weight by Drinking Water
https://www.everydayhealth.com/weight/can-you-lose-weight-by-drinking-water/

UAB — Debunking water myths: weight loss, calorie burn and more
https://www.uab.edu/news/youcanuse/item/4350-debunking-water-myths-weight-loss-calorie-burn-and-more

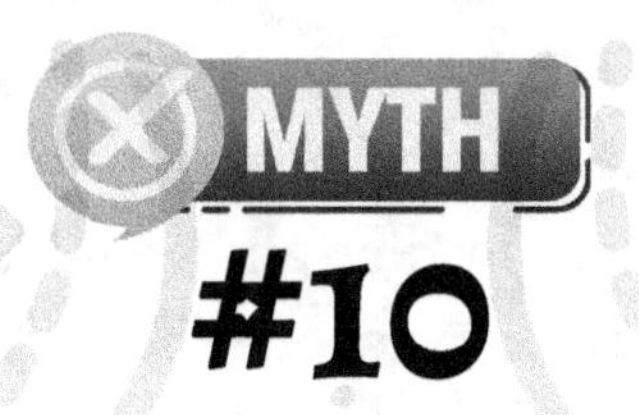

Weight loss supplements are effective

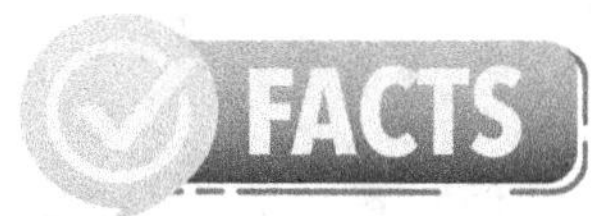

Supplements are not a magic solution and can have side effects.

The belief that weight loss supplements are effective solutions for shedding pounds is largely a myth. Many people turn to these products hoping for quick results, but the reality is more complex and often disappointing.

Most weight loss supplements on the market lack robust scientific evidence supporting their efficacy. For instance, the Mayo Clinic points out that many supplements haven't undergone rigorous clinical trials. Even when studies are conducted, they are often too small or too short to provide conclusive results. For example, a trial involving raspberry ketone showed minimal weight loss, but the trial's design prevents generalization to broader populations.

Moreover, the safety of these supplements is a significant concern. The FDA does not require supplements to be proven safe or effective before they are sold. This lack of regulation means that many supplements can contain harmful ingredients or contaminants. A survey reported by NutritionFacts.org found that dietary supplements cause about 50,000 adverse events annually, including serious conditions like liver and kidney damage.

Even FDA-approved weight loss medications, which undergo more stringent testing, come with potential side effects. For example, Qsymia and Contrave, both prescription medications, have been linked to side effects such as altered taste, insomnia, and increased risk of liver damage.

Ultimately, experts recommend a cautious approach to weight loss supplements. Registered dietitians and healthcare providers often emphasize that sustainable weight loss typically involves a balanced diet and regular physical activity rather than relying on supplements. It's also essential to consult with a healthcare provider before starting any new supplement, especially given the potential for harmful side effects and interactions with other medications.

For those considering weight loss supplements, it's critical to approach them with a healthy dose of skepticism and to prioritize safe, proven methods for weight management.

External links:

BarBend — The 10 Best Supplements for Weight Loss of 2024
https://barbend.com/best-supplements-for-weight-loss/

EverydayHealth.com — Top 5 FDA-Approved Weight Loss Pills: Full Review
https://www.everydayhealth.com/weight/best-weight-loss-pills-pros-cons-and-how-they-work/

Mayo Clinic — Dietary supplements for weight loss
https://www.mayoclinic.org/healthy-lifestyle/weight-loss/in-depth/weight-loss/art-20046409

NutritionFacts.org — The Safety of Weight-Loss Supplements
https://nutritionfacts.org/blog/the-safety-of-weight-loss-supplements/

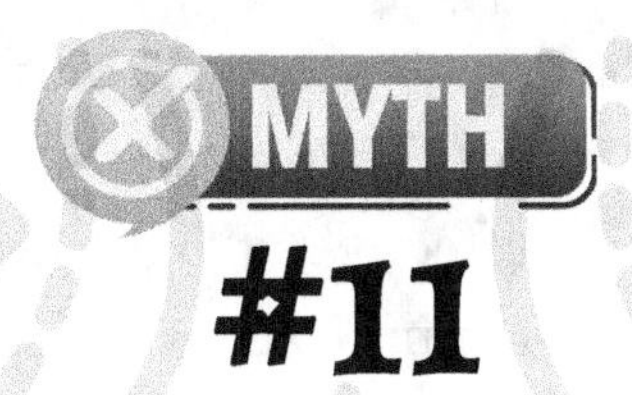

You can target fat loss in specific areas

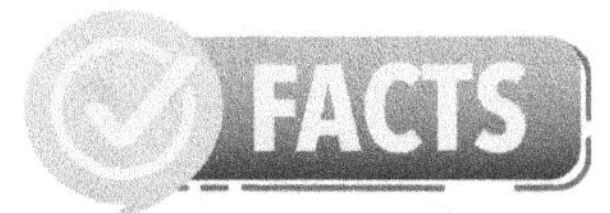

Spot reduction is a myth; fat loss occurs evenly throughout the body.

The idea that you can target fat loss in specific areas of the body, known as "spot reduction," is a common myth. Scientific research consistently shows that fat loss occurs evenly throughout the body, rather than being localized to specific areas targeted by exercise.

When we engage in physical activity, our bodies use stored fat as an energy source through a process called lipolysis. This process converts triglycerides from fat cells into free fatty acids and glycerol, which then travel through the bloodstream to be used as fuel by our muscles. Consequently, fat loss occurs across the entire body and is not limited to the area being exercised. This means that doing crunches or leg lifts alone will not specifically reduce belly or thigh fat.

Several studies support this view. For instance, a 2007 study published in "Medicine and Science in Sports and Exercise" found no significant fat loss in specific areas following a targeted resistance training program. Similarly, a 2013 study on leg exercises showed that while overall fat mass was reduced, there was no significant reduction in fat at the exercised body segment. These findings indicate that while targeted exercises can strengthen and tone muscles, they do not lead to localized fat loss.

Moreover, factors such as genetics, gender, and age play significant roles in determining where we store and lose fat. For example, women tend to store fat in their hips and thighs, while men often accumulate fat around the abdomen. These patterns are largely dictated by genetic and hormonal differences, making it difficult to control fat distribution through exercise alone.

Effective fat loss requires a holistic approach, including a balanced diet, regular cardiovascular exercise, and strength training. Cardiovascular exercises, such as running or cycling, are particularly effective at burning calories and promoting overall fat loss, while strength training helps build muscle, which increases metabolic rate and supports fat loss throughout the body.

In conclusion, the concept of spot reduction is a myth. Sustainable fat loss involves creating a calorie deficit through diet and exercise, leading to overall fat reduction rather than targeted fat loss in specific areas.

External links:

The University of Sydney — Spot reduction: why targeting weight loss to a specific area is a myth
https://www.sydney.edu.au/news-opinion/news/2023/11/07/spot-reduction--why-targeting-weight-loss-to-a-specific-area-is-.html

MiamiOH Sites — 2024 Reality Check: Effective Techniques for Belly Fat Loss
https://sites.miamioh.edu/student-healthy-life/2024/03/22/en-2024-reality-check-effective-techniques-for-belly-fat-loss/

Strength Zone Training — Spot Reduction: Real Science AND Exercise Myth
https://www.strengthzonetraining.com/spot-reduction-real-science-and-exercise-myth/

Yale Scientific — Targeted Fat Loss: Myth or Reality?
https://www.yalescientific.org/2011/04/targeted-fat-loss-myth-or-reality/

MiamiOH Sites — Top 5 Myths Debunked About Losing Belly Fat: What 2024 Research Shows
https://sites.miamioh.edu/student-healthy-life/2024/03/22/en-top-5-myths-debunked-about-losing-belly-fat-what-2024-research-shows/

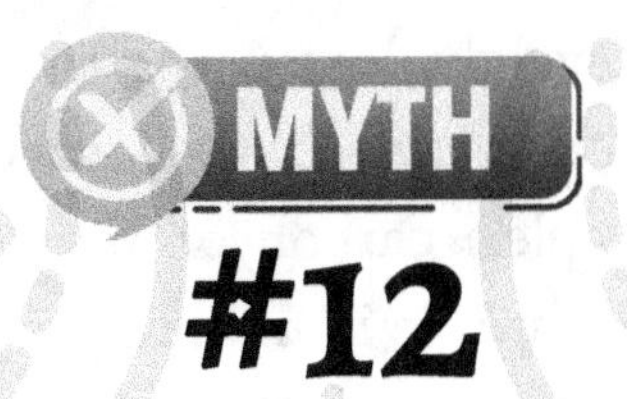

Eating small, frequent meals boosts metabolism

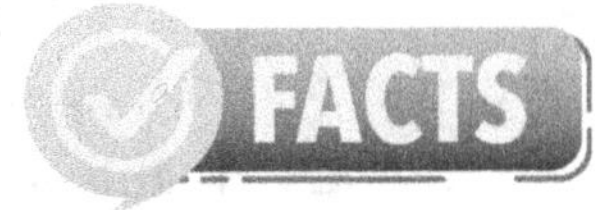

The frequency of meals doesn't boost metabolism significantly.

The belief that eating small, frequent meals boosts metabolism is a common myth. Scientific evidence shows that meal frequency does not significantly impact metabolic rate. The total amount of food consumed, rather than how often you eat, has a greater effect on your metabolism.

One key concept in this discussion is the thermic effect of food (TEF), which is the energy expenditure associated with digestion, absorption, and storage of nutrients. TEF typically accounts for about 10% of your total caloric intake, regardless of how those calories are distributed throughout the day. This means that eating six small meals or three large meals results in the same TEF, provided the total calorie intake is equal.

Research supports this finding. A study from the University of Ottawa found no significant difference in weight loss or metabolic rate between individuals who ate six meals a day and those who ate three. Similarly, another study concluded that switching from three to six meals per day did not enhance calorie burning or fat loss.

Furthermore, frequent eating can sometimes lead to increased overall calorie consumption. Smaller meals may not provide the same level of satiety as larger meals, potentially causing people to eat more overall. This can make it harder to control calorie intake, which is crucial for weight management.

Ultimately, what matters most for metabolism and weight loss is the total caloric intake and the nutritional quality of the food consumed. A balanced diet rich in whole foods, lean proteins, and complex carbohydrates is essential. Regular physical activity also plays a significant role in maintaining a healthy metabolism and promoting weight loss.

In summary, while eating small, frequent meals can help manage hunger and prevent overeating, it does not inherently boost metabolism. Focusing on overall dietary quality and caloric intake, along with regular exercise, is a more effective strategy for weight management.

⎋ External links:

SimpleHealthApp — Does Eating Small Frequent Meals Work For Weight Loss?
https://simple.life/blog/small-frequent-meals/

Discover Real Food in Texas — Does Eating Small, Frequent Meals Boost Your Metabolism? Expert Analysis and Facts
https://discover.texasrealfood.com/food-myth-buster/does-eating-small-frequent-meals-boost-your-metabolism

MDLinx — 5 myths about boosting metabolism debunked
https://www.mdlinx.com/article/5-myths-about-boosting-metabolism-debunked/7xtAhmM2AcH11x0G3O5Foh

MedlinePlus — Can you boost your metabolism?
https://medlineplus.gov/ency/patientinstructions/000893.htm

ShapeScale — Monday Myths – Eating Little And Often Will Boost Metabolis
https://shapescale.com/blog/monday-myths/myth-small-frequent-meals/

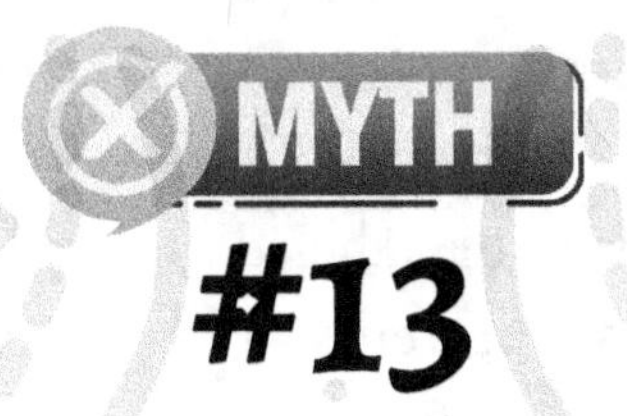

All-natural, organic, or gluten-free foods always lead to weight loss

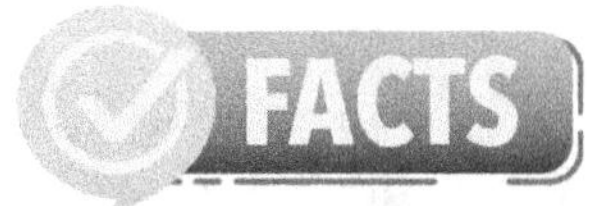

Organic or gluten-free foods are not necessarily lower in calories or better for weight loss.

The notion that all-natural, organic, or gluten-free foods inherently lead to weight loss is a common myth. While these labels may imply health benefits, they do not necessarily translate to lower calorie content or improved weight management.

Firstly, organic foods are grown without synthetic pesticides and fertilizers, which can have environmental and health benefits. However, they can still be high in calories, sugars, and fats, similar to their non-organic counterparts. For instance, organic cookies or chips may be perceived as healthier but often contain the same or even higher calorie content as regular versions due to added sugars and fats to enhance flavor and texture.

Similarly, gluten-free products are essential for individuals with celiac disease or non-celiac gluten sensitivity, but they are not inherently healthier for the general population. Many gluten-free foods compensate for the lack of gluten by adding extra sugar, fat, and sodium, which can increase the calorie content. A gluten-free cookie, for example, is still a cookie and can be just as high in calories as a regular one.

Moreover, the term "all-natural" is often used as a marketing tool and does not necessarily mean that the food is low in calories or beneficial for weight loss. Natural foods can include high-calorie ingredients like sugars and fats, and without proper portion control, they can contribute to weight gain just like any other food.

Effective weight management comes down to maintaining a balanced diet that controls calorie intake and includes a variety of nutrient-dense foods, regardless of whether they are organic, gluten-free, or labeled natural. Emphasizing whole foods like fruits, vegetables, lean proteins, and whole grains, along with regular physical activity, is a more reliable approach to achieving and maintaining a healthy weight.

In summary, while organic, gluten-free, and all-natural foods can be part of a healthy diet, they do not guarantee weight loss and should be consumed mindfully within the context of overall caloric and nutritional balance.

External links:

Cleveland Clinic — Can Gluten-Free Foods Help Aid Weight Loss?
https://health.clevelandclinic.org/the-surprising-truth-about-gluten-free-food-and-weight-loss

EverydayHealth.com — The Truth About Gluten: Myths and Facts
https://health.clevelandclinic.org/the-surprising-truth-about-gluten-free-food-and-weight-loss

Global News — Reality Check: Superfoods, organic food, paleo and gluten-free diets
https://globalnews.ca/news/2057186/reality-check-superfoods-organic-food-paleo-and-gluten-free-diets/

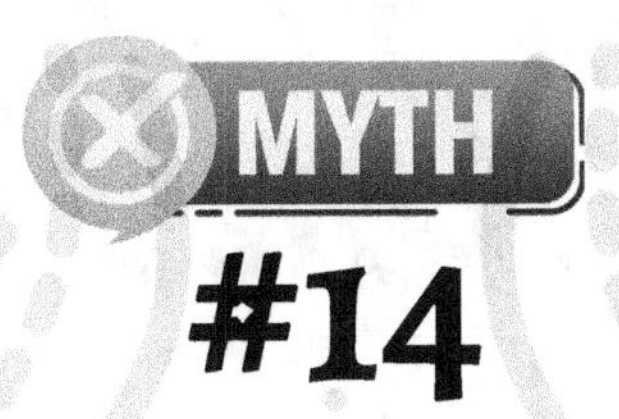

All smoothies are healthy and aid weight loss

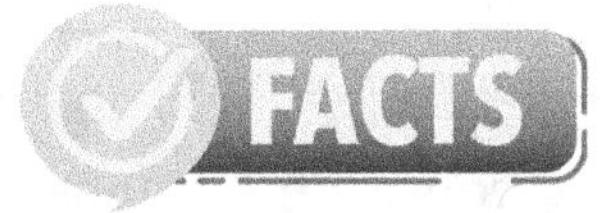

Not all smoothies are healthy; some contain high amounts of sugar.

The idea that all smoothies are inherently healthy and promote weight loss is a common misconception. While smoothies can be a convenient way to consume fruits and vegetables, not all smoothies are created equal, and some can be quite high in sugar and calories, which can hinder weight loss efforts.

Many commercially available smoothies and even some homemade versions can contain high amounts of added sugars and calorie-dense ingredients. For example, smoothies made with fruit juices, sweetened yogurts, or added sugars like honey and syrups can spike the calorie count significantly without providing much satiety. This is because liquid calories do not always make you feel as full as solid foods, leading to potential overeating later on.

Moreover, while fruits are nutritious, they naturally contain sugars, and when blended, they can lead to a high glycemic load, which might affect blood sugar levels. It's essential to balance smoothies with ingredients that provide protein and healthy fats, such as Greek yogurt, nuts, or seeds, to help maintain satiety and prevent blood sugar spikes.

Another issue with some smoothies is the loss of fiber. Whole fruits contain fiber that helps slow the absorption of sugar, but this fiber can be reduced or lost when fruits are juiced or over-blended. Fiber is crucial for maintaining digestive health and keeping you full longer, which is beneficial for weight management.

To make a healthier smoothie that supports weight loss, focus on whole, nutrient-dense ingredients. Use whole fruits instead of fruit juices, include plenty of vegetables, and add protein sources like unsweetened Greek yogurt or plant-based protein powders. Avoid adding sweeteners and opt for water or unsweetened almond milk as a base.

In summary, while smoothies can be a part of a healthy diet, it's important to be mindful of their ingredients. Not all smoothies are low in calories or sugar, and consuming high-sugar smoothies regularly can impede weight loss efforts. Balancing smoothies with protein, healthy fats, and fiber-rich ingredients can help make them a more effective tool for maintaining a healthy weight.

External links:

henryford.com — 10 Nutrition Myths About Weight Loss You Should Stop Believing
https://www.henryford.com/blog/2024/01/10-nutrition-myths

The Healthy — Weight Loss Smoothies That'll Help You Slim Down
https://www.thehealthy.com/weight-loss/weight-loss-smoothies-recipes/

All Nutritious — 10 Weight Loss Smoothies to Burn Fat
https://allnutritious.com/weight-loss-smoothies/

Simple Green Smoothies — 10 Best Fat-Burning Smoothies for Weight Loss
https://simplegreensmoothies.com/fat-burning-smoothie

Eat This Not That — Ways Drinking Smoothies Can Help You Lose Weight, Say Dietitians
https://www.eatthis.com/drinking-smoothies-weight-loss/

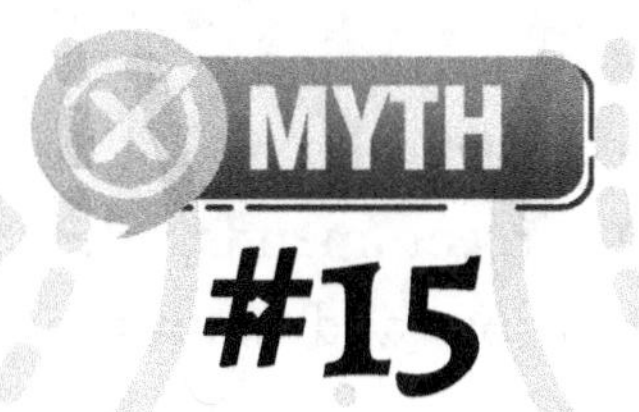

You need to be on a strict diet to lose weight

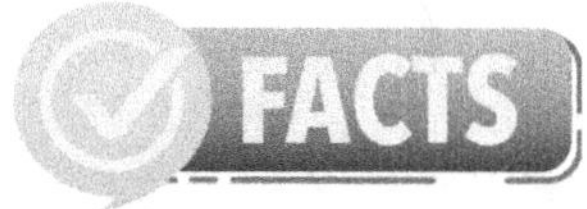

Balanced eating and portion control are key, not extreme dieting.

The belief that one must follow a strict diet to lose weight is a common myth. In reality, balanced eating and portion control are more effective and sustainable approaches to weight loss. Extreme diets often promise rapid results, but they can lead to nutritional deficiencies and are difficult to maintain in the long term.

A balanced diet emphasizes consuming a variety of nutrient-dense foods, including fruits, vegetables, whole grains, lean proteins, and healthy fats. This approach ensures that your body receives all the essential nutrients it needs to function optimally. According to the Mayo Clinic, a flexible and balanced diet plan, which includes a wide range of foods and allows occasional treats, is more sustainable and effective for long-term weight loss and health maintenance.

In contrast, restrictive diets often eliminate entire food groups or significantly cut calories, leading to potential nutrient deficiencies and a negative relationship with food. Such diets can cause cycles of extreme restriction followed by periods of overeating, which can disrupt metabolism and hinder weight loss efforts. A healthy diet, on the other hand, focuses on moderation, allowing for occasional indulgences without guilt.

Research supports that a balanced diet combined with portion control is effective for weight management. By consuming a variety of whole foods in appropriate portions, you can maintain a healthy weight and reduce the risk of obesity and related chronic diseases. Studies have shown that diets rich in fruits, vegetables, whole grains, and lean proteins are associated with lower risks of heart disease, diabetes, and certain cancers.

Moreover, incorporating regular physical activity into your routine enhances the benefits of a balanced diet. Exercise not only helps burn calories but also improves overall health and well-being. The Mayo Clinic recommends at least 30 minutes of physical activity daily to support weight loss and maintain a healthy lifestyle.

In summary, you do not need to be on a strict diet to lose weight. A balanced diet, portion control, and regular physical activity are key to achieving and maintaining a healthy weight sustainably. This approach promotes overall health and well-being, making it a more practical and enjoyable path to weight loss.

⤴ External links:

Mayo Clinic — The Mayo Clinic Diet: A weight-loss program for life
https://www.mayoclinic.org/healthy-lifestyle/weight-loss/in-depth/mayo-clinic-diet/art-20045460

Mayo Clinic — Weight loss: Choosing a diet that's right for you
https://www.mayoclinic.org/healthy-lifestyle/weight-loss/in-depth/weight-loss/art-20048466

Lean Body Goals — Healthy Diet vs. Dieting: Understanding the Difference
https://leanbodygoals.com/healthy-diet-vs-dieting-understanding-the-difference/

Essential Sports Nutrition — Balanced Diet vs Fad Diets: What's the Difference?
https://essentialsportsnutrition.com/blogs/news/balanced-diet-vs-fad-diets-whats-the-difference

My Shapa — Balanced Diet vs. Fad Diets: Which is Better for Sustainable Weight Loss?
https://home.myshapa.com/balanced-diet-vs-fad-diets/

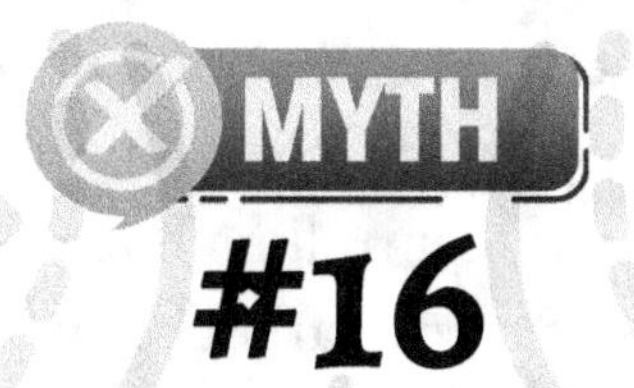

Eating fat-free or low-fat foods is better

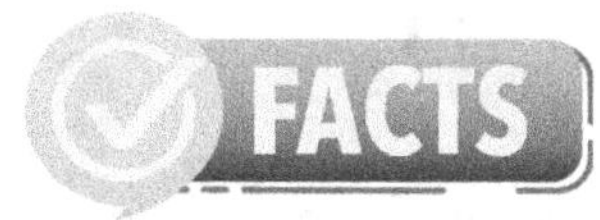

Low-fat or fat-free foods can be high in sugar and calories.

The idea that eating fat-free or low-fat foods is better for weight loss and overall health is a widespread myth. In reality, many low-fat or fat-free products are often high in sugar and calories, which can counteract the benefits of reducing fat intake.

When manufacturers remove fat from food products, they often add sugar and other additives to maintain taste and texture. This can result in foods that are low in fat but high in sugar and calories. For instance, low-fat yogurts and snacks frequently contain added sugars to compensate for the flavor lost when fat is removed. This can lead to an increased calorie intake and may contribute to weight gain rather than weight loss.

Moreover, the perception that low-fat foods are healthier can lead people to consume larger portions, underestimating their calorie content. Research indicates that people tend to eat more of a product if they believe it is healthy, which can result in consuming more calories than intended.

Fats are an essential part of a balanced diet, providing satiety and supporting various bodily functions. Healthy fats, such as those found in avocados, nuts, and olive oil, can help maintain heart health and should be included in a balanced diet. These fats can help keep you full longer, reducing the likelihood of overeating.

For effective weight management and overall health, it is crucial to focus on a balanced diet that includes a variety of nutrients rather than simply eliminating fats. Emphasizing whole, unprocessed foods, controlling portion sizes, and maintaining a balanced intake of fats, proteins, and carbohydrates is more beneficial than relying on low-fat or fat-free products that may be misleading.

In conclusion, while low-fat or fat-free foods might seem like a healthier choice, they can often be high in sugar and calories, undermining weight loss efforts. A balanced diet that includes healthy fats is essential for long-term health and effective weight management.

External links:

Houston Methodist Leading Medicine — Don't Be Fooled by Low-Fat Foods
https://www.houstonmethodist.org/blog/articles/2020/jan/dont-be-fooled-by-low-fat-foods/

Cleveland Clinic — Which Is Worse for You: Fat or Sugar?
https://health.clevelandclinic.org/which-is-worse-for-you-fat-or-sugar

UChicago Medicine — Is full-fat food better than low-fat or fat-free food?
https://www.uchicagomedicine.org/forefront/gastrointestinal-articles/2023/july/which-are-healthier-low-fat-or-full-fat-foods

MedXpress — Truthful yet misleading packaging: Consumers falsely believe that low fat means less sugar
https://medicalxpress.com/news/2023-06-truthful-packaging-consumers-falsely-fat.html

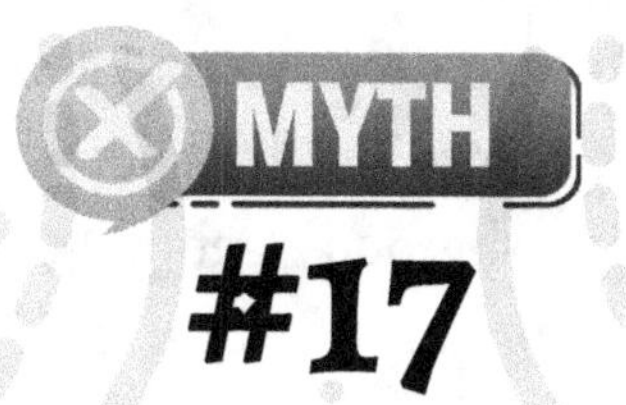

Fasting is the best way to lose weight

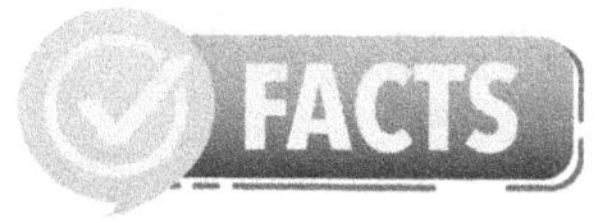

Fasting can lead to muscle loss and nutritional deficiencies.

The notion that fasting is the best way to lose weight is a common myth. While fasting can lead to weight loss, it also poses significant risks, including muscle loss and nutritional deficiencies.

Fasting, particularly prolonged or extreme fasting, can lead to the body breaking down muscle tissue for energy. This is because, in the absence of food, the body may not receive enough protein to maintain muscle mass, leading to muscle degradation. Preserving muscle mass is crucial as muscles help maintain metabolic rate, and losing muscle can slow down metabolism, making it harder to lose weight in the long run.

Additionally, fasting can result in nutritional deficiencies. By severely restricting calorie intake, individuals may not consume adequate vitamins and minerals necessary for overall health. This can lead to issues such as electrolyte imbalances, heart arrhythmias, dizziness, dehydration, and other health problems. For instance, electrolytes like sodium and potassium are essential for heart and muscle function, and their imbalance can cause serious health issues.

Moreover, extreme fasting can trigger what is known as "starvation mode," where the body slows down its metabolism to conserve energy, making weight loss more challenging. It can also increase the likelihood of binge eating once the fast ends, as the body tries to compensate for the calorie deficit, potentially leading to a cycle of fasting and overeating.

A more sustainable and healthier approach to weight loss involves balanced eating and regular physical activity. This includes consuming a variety of nutrient-dense foods in appropriate portions, ensuring the body gets all the essential nutrients it needs to function properly. Regular exercise helps maintain muscle mass and boosts metabolism, contributing to more effective and lasting weight loss.

In conclusion, while fasting can lead to weight loss, it is not the best approach due to the risks of muscle loss and nutritional deficiencies. A balanced diet combined with regular exercise is a more effective and sustainable strategy for achieving and maintaining a healthy weight.

External links:

LifeMD™ — Intermittent Fasting Myths
https://lifemd.com/learn/intermittent-fasting-myths

Beaumont — Fasting for Weight Loss | Safety Tips and More
https://www.beaumont.org/services/weight-loss/what-is-fasting

MyFitnessPal Blog — Is Fasting Really a Safe Way to Lose Weight?
https://blog.myfitnesspal.com/is-fasting-really-a-safe-way-to-lose-weight/

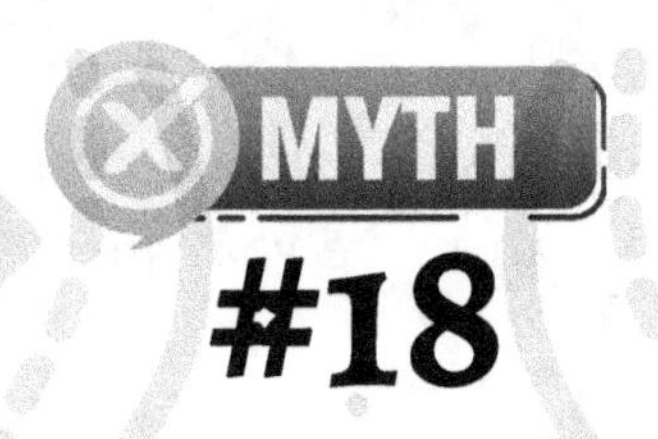

You have to give up your favorite foods to lose weight

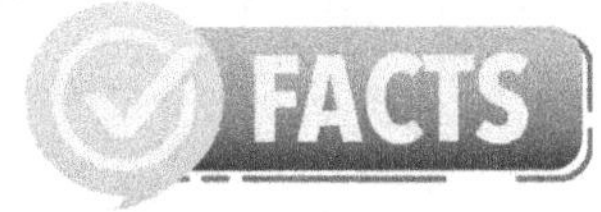

You can enjoy your favorite foods in moderation as part of a healthy diet.

The belief that you need to give up your favorite foods to lose weight is a common myth. In reality, you can enjoy your favorite foods in moderation as part of a healthy diet and still achieve your weight loss goals. This approach is more sustainable and prevents the feelings of deprivation that often accompany restrictive diets.

Moderation and portion control are key strategies for including your favorite foods in a weight loss plan. By paying attention to portion sizes and practicing mindful eating, you can savor small amounts of your favorite treats without overindulging. Mindful eating involves savoring each bite and being aware of your body's hunger and fullness cues, which can help you feel satisfied with less food.

Incorporating your favorite foods in a balanced diet can also help maintain long-term dietary adherence. For instance, allowing yourself occasional indulgences can prevent the urge to binge on restricted items later. This balanced approach aligns with the principles of various successful diets, such as the Mediterranean diet, which emphasizes nutrient-rich foods without strict calorie counting.

Moreover, making healthier versions of your favorite dishes can allow you to enjoy them more frequently. Simple substitutions, like using whole grains instead of refined grains or baking instead of frying, can make your meals healthier without sacrificing flavor.

Ultimately, the key to successful weight loss is not eliminating favorite foods but integrating them into a balanced and varied diet. This strategy not only supports weight management but also promotes a healthier relationship with food, ensuring that your dietary changes are sustainable over the long term.

⬈ External links:

Mayo Clinic Diet — Eat what you love and still lose weight
https://diet.mayoclinic.org/us/blog/2022/eat-what-you-love-and-still-lose-weight/

Lorie Eber Wellness Coaching — Can I Lose Weight Without Giving Up Favorite Foods?
https://lorieeberwellnesscoaching.com/can-i-lose-weight-without-giving-up-favorite-foods/

Chcf's Resource — Can you eat junk food and still lose weight?
https://www.chefsresource.com/can-you-eat-junk-food-and-still-lose-weight/

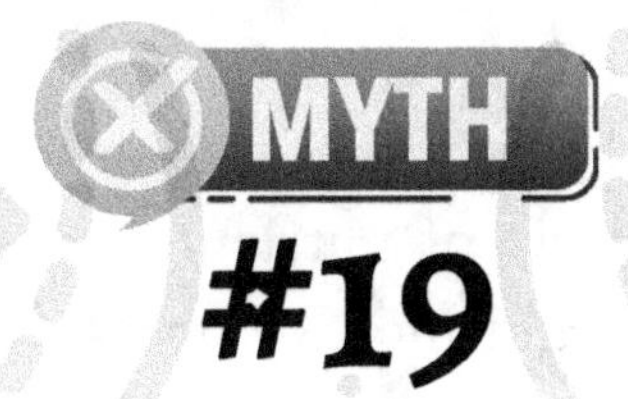

Dairy products cause weight gain

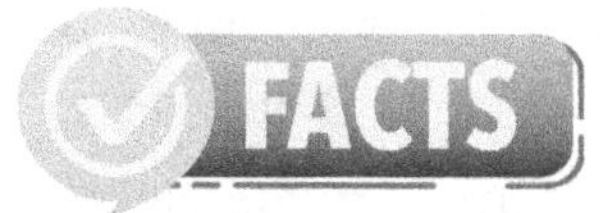

Dairy products can be part of a balanced diet and do not necessarily cause weight gain.

The belief that dairy products cause weight gain is a widespread myth. In reality, dairy products can be part of a balanced diet and do not necessarily lead to weight gain. In fact, they can even support weight loss and overall health.

Dairy products, such as milk, cheese, and yogurt, provide essential nutrients like calcium, vitamin D, and protein. These nutrients are vital for maintaining bone health, muscle function, and overall metabolic processes. Studies have shown that the inclusion of dairy in a balanced diet does not correlate with weight gain. On the contrary, higher dairy calcium intake has been associated with improved weight loss and reduced body fat.

One of the reasons dairy products are beneficial for weight management is their role in promoting satiety. The fat content in dairy helps extend feelings of fullness, which can reduce overall calorie intake. This satiety effect is particularly important for those looking to control their appetite and avoid overeating.

Moreover, the protein in dairy products can help build and maintain lean muscle mass, which is crucial for a healthy metabolism. More muscle mass means your body burns more calories at rest, aiding in weight loss efforts. Studies have indicated that individuals who consume dairy as part of their diet tend to have better outcomes in preserving muscle mass and reducing fat mass compared to those who do not.

It's also worth noting that cutting out dairy without a medical reason, such as lactose intolerance or a dairy allergy, might not be beneficial. Instead, focusing on portion control and incorporating a variety of nutrient-dense foods, including dairy, can contribute to a healthier and more sustainable weight loss journey.

In summary, dairy products do not inherently cause weight gain and can be included in a balanced diet to support weight management and overall health. The key is moderation and ensuring that dairy is part of a varied and nutrient-rich diet.

⎋ External links:

iowafarmbureau.com — Busting nutrition myths: How to eat healthier
https://www.iowafarmbureau.com/Article/Busting-nutrition-myths-How-to-eat-healthier-in-2024

Got Milk — Busting Myths About Dairy and Weight Gain
https://www.gotmilk.com/busting-myth-about-dairy-and-weight-gain/

Eat This Not That — Will Cutting Out Dairy Help You Lose Weight?
https://www.eatthis.com/no-dairy-weight-loss/

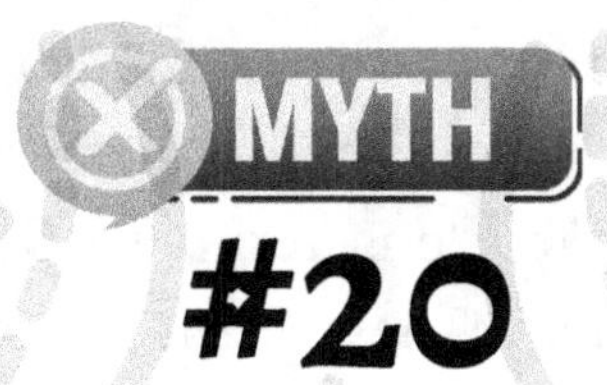

All 'low-carb' diets are the sam

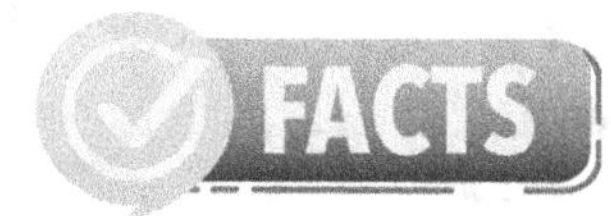

Different low-carb diets have different impacts and are not all equally effective.

The belief that all low-carb diets are the same is a common misconception. In reality, different low-carb diets have distinct impacts and are not equally effective for everyone. The key differences lie in their specific food compositions, nutrient quality, and overall health benefits.

Low-carb diets generally focus on reducing carbohydrate intake, but the extent and type of carbohydrates allowed can vary significantly. For instance, the ketogenic (keto) diet is one of the most restrictive, aiming to put the body into a state of ketosis where it burns fat for fuel instead of carbohydrates. This diet typically involves consuming fewer than 50 grams of carbs per day and emphasizes high fat intake. While keto can lead to rapid weight loss and improvements in certain health markers, it can be challenging to maintain long-term and may cause initial side effects like the "keto flu.

On the other hand, diets like Atkins and Paleo also reduce carbs but have different approaches and restrictions. The Atkins diet is phased, starting with very low carbs and gradually reintroducing them, which can be more sustainable for some people. Paleo focuses on foods presumed to be available to early humans, such as meat, fish, fruits, vegetables, nuts, and seeds, while excluding processed foods, grains, and dairy. This can make Paleo less restrictive in terms of carb intake compared to keto, but it still emphasizes high protein and fat from natural sources.

Moreover, research has highlighted the importance of the quality of foods in these diets. Plant-based low-carb diets, which emphasize proteins and fats from vegetables, nuts, and seeds, have shown better long-term weight maintenance compared to animal-based low-carb diets. These plant-based diets are associated with slower weight gain over time and improved metabolic health, emphasizing the role of food quality over simply reducing carb intake.

In conclusion, not all low-carb diets are created equal. Their effectiveness and health impacts can vary widely depending on their specific guidelines and the quality of foods consumed. It is crucial to choose a diet that fits individual health needs, preferences, and lifestyle for sustainable weight management and overall well-being.

External links:

EverydayHealth.com — For Low-Carb Diets, Quality of Food, Not Just Quantity, Is Key to Long-Term Weight Loss
https://www.everydayhealth.com/diet-nutritrion/best-low-carb-diet-for-keeping-weight-off-according-to-new-harvard-study/

Harvard Gazette — Plant-based low-carb diet best for long-term weight loss
https://news.harvard.edu/gazette/story/2024/01/looking-for-the-best-low-carb-diet-plant-based-wins-again/

Iowa Clinic — The Most Popular Low-Carb Diets, Compared
https://www.iowaclinic.com/primary-care/specialties/internal-medicine/low-carb-diet-comparison/

The Nutrition Source — Diet Review: Ketogenic Diet for Weight Loss
https://nutritionsource.hsph.harvard.edu/healthy-weight/diet-reviews/ketogenic-diet/

MYTH #21: You need to eat only 'clean' foods to lose weight

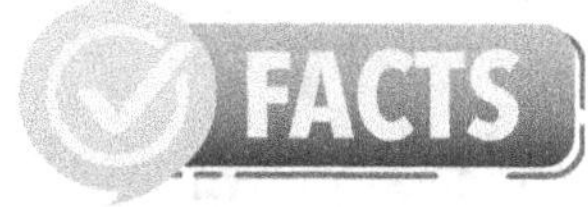

Clean eating is good, but balance and moderation are key.

The myth that you need to eat only "clean" foods to lose weight is misleading. While clean eating, which involves consuming whole, unprocessed foods, can contribute to better health, balance and moderation are crucial for sustainable weight loss.

Clean eating emphasizes whole foods like fruits, vegetables, lean proteins, and whole grains while avoiding processed foods. This approach can help reduce intake of added sugars, unhealthy fats, and excess sodium, which are often found in processed foods. However, labeling foods as "clean" or "unclean" can lead to an unhealthy mindset, where certain foods are viewed as inherently bad, potentially fostering guilt and disordered eating behaviors. It's important to have a flexible approach that allows for occasional indulgences without guilt.

Research shows that focusing solely on clean eating can sometimes lead to nutrient deficiencies if the diet becomes too restrictive. For example, completely eliminating processed foods might reduce essential nutrients that fortified foods can provide. Moreover, strict clean eating can lead to social isolation and stress about food choices, which are not conducive to long-term health or weight management.

Balance and moderation are key to a sustainable diet. Incorporating a variety of foods, including occasional treats, helps maintain a healthy relationship with food and ensures a broad spectrum of nutrients. A diet rich in minimally processed foods, such as those found in the Mediterranean diet, which includes fruits, vegetables, whole grains, nuts, and healthy fats, has been shown to support weight loss and overall health without the need for extreme restrictions.

In conclusion, while clean eating has its benefits, a balanced diet that includes a variety of foods in moderation is more effective and sustainable for weight loss. Avoiding an all-or-nothing mindset and allowing yourself flexibility can help you maintain healthy eating habits in the long term.

↗ External links:

Foodborne Wellness - The clean eating myth: how "clean eating" challenges a healthy mindset.
https://foodbornewellness.com/clean-eating-weight-loss/

Nutrition Letter - Busting Weight Loss Myths
https://www.nutritionletter.tufts.edu/healthy-eating/busting-weight-loss-myths-2/

Eat This Not That - 7 Clean Eating Habits for Weight Loss, According to Dietitians
https://www.eatthis.com/clean-eating-habits-for-weight-loss/

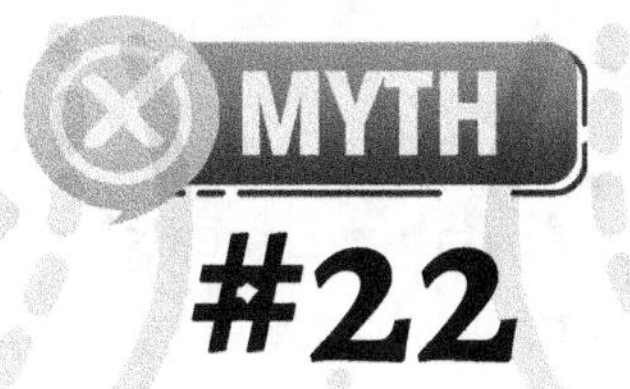

Exercise makes you hungrier and leads to weight gain

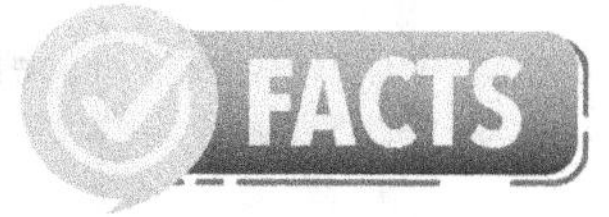

Exercise can increase appetite, but mindful eating can help manage hunger.

The belief that exercise makes you hungrier and leads to weight gain is a common myth. While exercise can increase appetite, managing hunger through mindful eating can help prevent unwanted weight gain.

Firstly, moderate exercise tends to suppress appetite temporarily by increasing levels of peptide YY, a hormone that reduces hunger. This effect can last for several hours post-exercise, helping to control immediate post-workout hunger pangs. Additionally, studies have shown that moderate exercise does not lead to compensatory overeating, meaning that people do not necessarily eat more after exercising than they would if they remained sedentary.

On the other hand, strength training and high-intensity workouts can significantly increase appetite, as they cause more muscle damage that requires repair and energy. This increased energy demand can lead to a heightened feeling of hunger. However, this does not automatically translate into weight gain if managed properly. Consuming nutrient-dense foods and maintaining a balanced diet can help offset the increased hunger without leading to excessive calorie intake.

Moreover, initial weight gain from exercise can often be attributed to factors other than fat gain. For example, water retention due to glycogen storage in muscles can cause a temporary increase in weight. As your body adapts to regular exercise, this water weight typically decreases. Furthermore, gaining muscle mass, which is denser than fat, might show up as weight gain on the scale but actually represents a healthier body composition.

It's also important to consider the quality of calories consumed. Overeating calorie-dense, nutrient-poor foods in response to increased hunger can negate the benefits of exercise. Instead, focusing on balanced meals that include lean proteins, healthy fats, and complex carbohydrates can help manage hunger effectively.

In conclusion, while exercise can increase appetite, it does not necessarily lead to weight gain if mindful eating practices are employed. By understanding and managing post-exercise hunger, individuals can enjoy the benefits of exercise without the fear of unwanted weight gain. For more detailed guidance, consulting with a nutritionist or a fitness professional can be beneficial.

External links:

Verywell Fit — How Exercise Affects Appetite and Hunger
https://www.verywellfit.com/how-exercise-affects-appetite-5218713

Cleveland Clinic — I Just Started Exercising — Why Am I Gaining Weight?
https://health.clevelandclinic.org/just-started-exercising-gaining-weight

Anytime Fitness — 5 Reasons You're Gaining Weight While Working Out
https://www.anytimefitness.com/ccc/ask-a-coach/revealed-the-top-reasons-you-may-be-gaining-weight-while-working-out/

Verywell Fit — Why You Might Be Gaining Weight After Working Out
https://www.verywellfit.com/i-just-started-exercising-why-am-i-gaining-weight-1231585

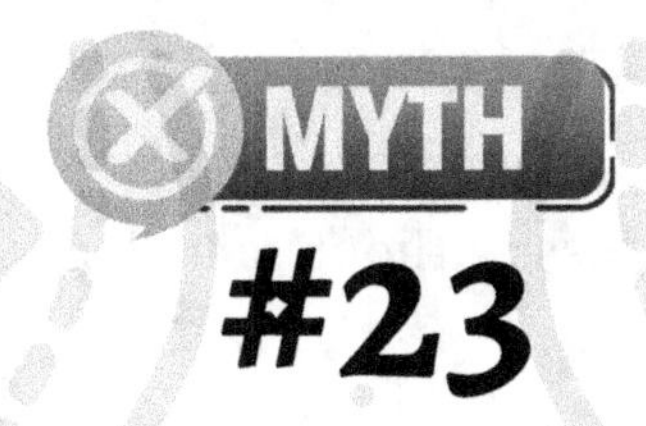

Cutting out entire food groups is necessary for weight loss

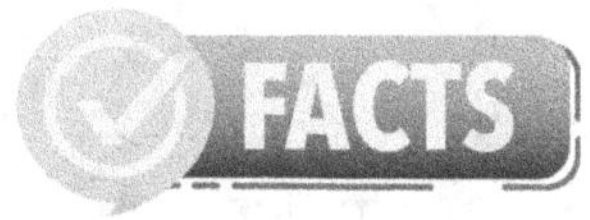

Eliminating entire food groups can lead to nutritional deficiencies.

Cutting out entire food groups is often perceived as a quick way to lose weight, but this approach can lead to significant nutritional deficiencies and isn't sustainable for long-term health. Instead of eliminating whole categories of food, focusing on a balanced diet that includes a variety of nutrients is crucial.

Elimination diets, such as those excluding carbs, fats, or dairy, can initially result in weight loss due to reduced calorie intake. However, these diets can deprive the body of essential nutrients. For example, carbohydrates are a primary energy source and provide necessary fiber and B vitamins, while dairy products offer calcium and vitamin D, crucial for bone health.

Moreover, fad diets that eliminate food groups are typically difficult to maintain and often result in weight regain once normal eating patterns are resumed. This cycle can negatively impact metabolism and make weight management even more challenging in the long run. Such restrictive diets can also lead to feelings of deprivation and increased cravings, making it harder to stick to healthy eating habits.

A more effective approach is to choose healthier options within each food group. For instance, opt for whole grains over processed grains, and include a variety of fruits, vegetables, lean proteins, and healthy fats in your diet. This strategy not only supports weight loss but also ensures you receive a broad spectrum of nutrients essential for overall health.

For those considering dietary changes, consulting with a healthcare provider or dietitian is advisable. They can provide personalized guidance and help develop a balanced eating plan that supports weight loss without sacrificing nutritional adequacy.

In summary, while cutting out entire food groups might seem like an effective weight-loss strategy, it can lead to nutritional deficiencies and is not sustainable. A balanced diet with a variety of nutrient-dense foods is the best approach for long-term health and weight management.

↗ External links:

Michigan Medicine — Elimination Diets: Dietary Restrictions and Weight Loss
https://www.michiganmedicine.org/health-lab/can-elimination-diet-help-you-lose-weight

BistroMD — Why You Should Not Cut Food Groups for Weight Loss
https://www.bistromd.com/blogs/weight-loss/why-its-not-good-to-cut-out-entire-food-groups-for-weight-loss

Cleveland Clinic — Fad Diets: What They Are and Are They Healthy
https://health.clevelandclinic.org/fad-diets

Health & Wellbeing — Why Cutting Out Food Groups Could Be Harming Your Health
https://www.healthwellbeing.com/why-cutting-out-food-groups-could-be-harming-your-health/

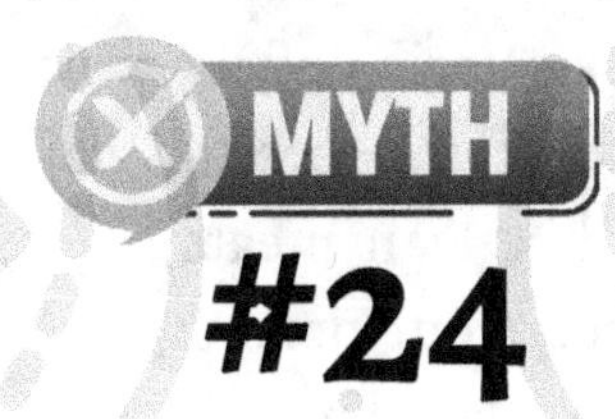

Protein shakes are essential for weight loss

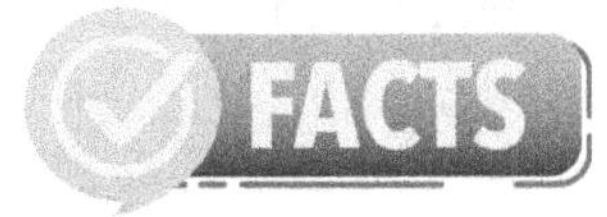

Protein shakes can be helpful but are not essential for weight loss.

The idea that protein shakes are essential for weight loss is a myth. While they can be helpful, they are not necessary for achieving weight loss goals.

Protein shakes can aid in weight loss by providing a convenient source of protein, which helps with muscle building and repair, and increases metabolism due to the thermic effect of food. Protein is more satiating compared to carbohydrates and fats, which can help reduce overall calorie intake throughout the day. This reduction in caloric intake is a key factor in weight loss.

However, relying solely on protein shakes for weight loss can have drawbacks. Protein shakes often lack the essential nutrients found in whole foods, such as fiber, vitamins, and minerals. This can lead to nutrient deficiencies if they are used to replace whole meals consistently. Additionally, some protein shakes contain added sugars and other additives that can contribute to a higher calorie intake, counteracting weight loss efforts.

Furthermore, the sustainability of a diet heavily reliant on protein shakes is questionable. Many people may find it difficult to maintain such a diet long-term due to taste fatigue and the social aspect of eating solid meals. A balanced diet incorporating a variety of whole foods is generally more effective and sustainable for long-term weight management.

To effectively lose weight, it is important to maintain a calorie deficit, which can be achieved by consuming fewer calories than you burn through daily activities and exercise. Including protein-rich foods like lean meats, eggs, dairy, legumes, and nuts in your diet can help you meet your protein needs without solely relying on shakes. Combining this with regular physical activity and healthy eating habits is the best approach for sustained weight loss and overall health.

In conclusion, while protein shakes can be a useful tool for weight loss, they are not essential. A balanced diet rich in whole foods, combined with regular exercise, is the most effective strategy for achieving and maintaining weight loss.

⬈ External links:

Verywell Fit — Protein Shakes for Weight Loss: Is a Protein Shake Diet Safe?
https://www.verywellfit.com/can-i-lose-weight-with-weight-loss-shakes-3496392

Mayo Clinic — Protein shakes: Good for weight loss?
https://www.mayoclinic.org/healthy-lifestyle/weight-loss/expert-answers/protein-shakes/faq-20058335

Cleveland Clinic — How Much Protein To Eat To Lose Weight
https://health.clevelandclinic.org/how-much-protein-to-eat-to-lose-weight

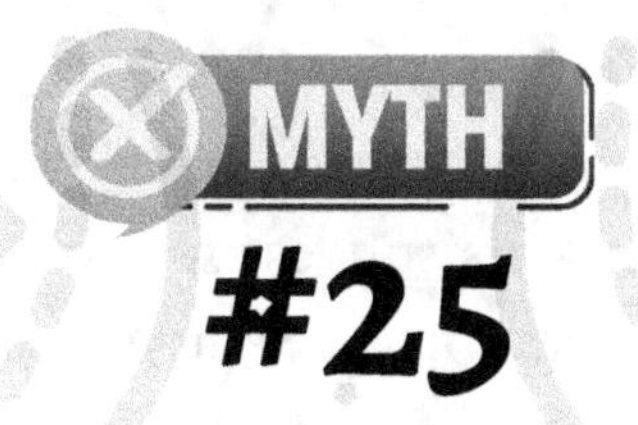

Eating more frequently increases metabolism

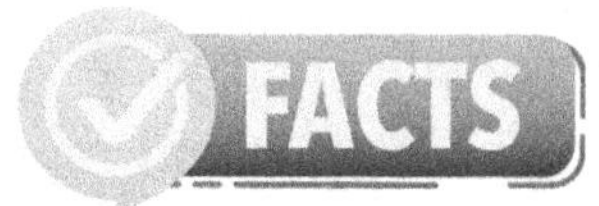

Increasing meal frequency doesn't significantly impact metabolism.

The myth that eating more frequently increases metabolism and aids in weight loss is widespread but not supported by scientific evidence. While the idea behind this myth is that frequent meals can boost your metabolism by increasing the thermic effect of food (TEF)—the energy expenditure required for digestion—research shows this effect is minimal and does not significantly impact overall metabolism.

The TEF does contribute to daily calorie expenditure, but it accounts for only about 10% of total energy expenditure, regardless of meal frequency. Therefore, eating more frequently does not lead to a proportionally higher metabolic rate. Studies comparing different meal frequencies have found no significant difference in metabolic rate or weight loss between those who eat more frequently and those who do not.

Moreover, the impact of meal frequency on weight management is more related to appetite control and dietary adherence than to metabolism. Eating more often can help some people manage hunger better and avoid overeating during meals. However, this does not translate to a metabolic advantage. A 2010 study in the British Journal of Nutrition found no significant weight loss difference between groups eating three meals per day and those eating three meals plus three snacks, provided total calorie intake was the same.

Additionally, the sustainability of frequent eating patterns can be challenging. It requires careful planning and portion control to avoid excessive calorie intake, which could counteract weight loss efforts. Experts suggest focusing on overall dietary quality and balanced meals rather than meal frequency to support weight management and metabolic health.

In conclusion, while eating more frequently may help some individuals control hunger and maintain a balanced diet, it does not significantly boost metabolism or enhance weight loss. The key to effective weight management is maintaining a calorie deficit through a balanced diet and regular physical activity, regardless of how meals are spaced throughout the day.

External links:

Livestrong.com — Does Eating Every Three Hours Really Raise Metabolism?
https://www.livestrong.com/article/410350-does-eating-every-three-hours-really-raise-metabolism/

MedlinePlus — Can you boost your metabolism?
https://medlineplus.gov/ency/patientinstructions/000893.htm

EliteFTS — Does Eating More Frequently Boost My Metabolism?
https://www.elitefts.com/education/does-eating-more-frequently-boost-my-metabolism/

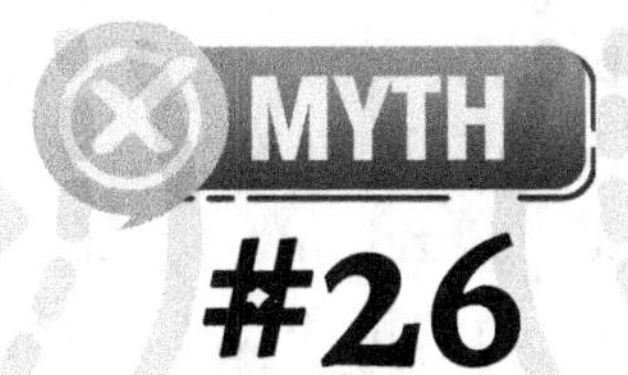

Drinking green tea melts fat away

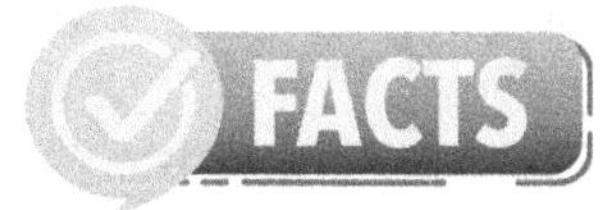

Green tea has health benefits but won't melt fat away.

The myth that drinking green tea melts fat away is not supported by scientific evidence. While green tea does offer several health benefits, it is not a magic solution for weight loss.

Green tea is rich in antioxidants, particularly catechins, which have been shown to provide various health benefits, including reducing inflammation and lowering the risk of heart disease. However, its impact on fat loss is minimal. Studies suggest that while green tea can slightly boost metabolism and increase fat oxidation, these effects are not significant enough to cause substantial weight loss on their own.

One study found that fat oxidation rates were about 17% higher in healthy men after consuming green tea extracts compared to a placebo, but this effect was modest and the study size was small, indicating that more research is needed to confirm these findings. Additionally, any increase in metabolism due to green tea is not sufficient to "melt fat away." Instead, the benefits are more related to overall health improvements rather than dramatic changes in body fat.

Experts emphasize that fat loss cannot be attributed to consuming or eliminating any single food or drink. Effective weight loss requires a combination of a balanced diet, regular exercise, and maintaining a caloric deficit. Green tea can be a part of a healthy diet, particularly if it replaces higher-calorie beverages, but it should not be relied upon as the primary method for weight loss.

In summary, while green tea is beneficial for health and can contribute to a slight increase in fat oxidation, it will not cause significant fat loss on its own. For effective weight management, focus on a comprehensive approach that includes a healthy diet, regular physical activity, and lifestyle changes.

External links:

India Today — Does green tea help in reducing belly fat?
https://www.indiatoday.in/health/story/does-green-tea-help-in-reducing-belly-fat-1948664-2022-05-12

CureJoy — Does Green Tea Burn Fat?
https://curejoy.com/content/does-green-tea-burn-fat/

Counting calories is the only way to lose weight

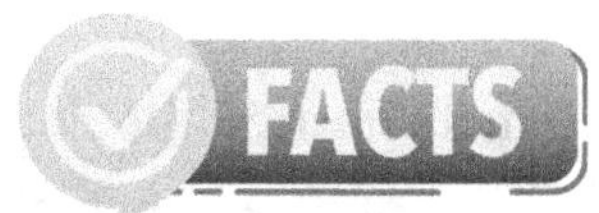

Counting calories can be helpful, but overall nutrition quality is more important.

The common belief that counting calories is the only effective way to lose weight is an oversimplification. While monitoring calorie intake can help some people manage their weight, focusing solely on calories ignores the complex ways our bodies process food and regulate weight.

Calorie counting is based on the principle of "calories in, calories out," which suggests that to lose weight, one must consume fewer calories than they expend. However, this method does not account for the body's adaptive mechanisms. When calorie intake is reduced, the body adjusts by slowing down the metabolism and altering hormone levels, making it harder to lose weight over time and easier to regain it.

Moreover, not all calories are equal in terms of nutrition and how they affect the body. For instance, 180 calories from nuts and 180 calories from pizza are processed differently. Nuts are high in fiber and healthy fats, which are absorbed more slowly and can help you feel full longer, whereas the refined carbohydrates in pizza can lead to rapid spikes and crashes in blood sugar, increasing hunger shortly after eating.

Quality of nutrition plays a crucial role in weight management. Whole foods like vegetables, fruits, lean proteins, and whole grains provide essential nutrients that support overall health and can help regulate appetite and energy levels more effectively than processed foods high in sugar and unhealthy fats. Additionally, these whole foods can positively influence gut health, inflammation, and hormonal balance, all of which are important for maintaining a healthy weight.

In conclusion, while counting calories can be a useful tool for some, it is not the only or the most effective approach for everyone. Emphasizing overall nutrition quality and understanding the body's complex responses to food can lead to more sustainable and healthful weight management strategies. For long-term success, a balanced diet rich in whole foods and a healthy lifestyle are key.

⬈ External links:

MedXpress — It's time to bust the 'calories in, calories out' weight-loss myth
https://medicalxpress.com/news/2023-06-calories-weight-loss-myth.html

The University of Sydney — It's time to bust the 'calories in, calories out' weight-loss myth
https://www.sydney.edu.au/news-opinion/news/2023/07/05/its-time-to-bust-the-calories-in-calories-out-weight-loss-myth.html

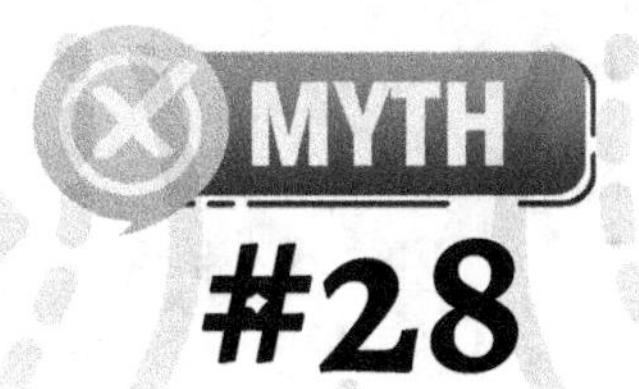

Weight loss is just about willpower

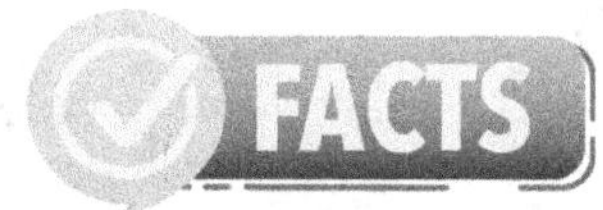

Weight loss involves more than just willpower; it's about habits and environment.

The myth that weight loss is purely a matter of willpower is both pervasive and misleading. The reality is that successful weight management involves a complex interplay of various factors, including habits, environment, psychology, and biology.

Firstly, while willpower does play a role in making healthy choices, it is not the sole driver of weight loss. Dr. Donald Hensrud from the Mayo Clinic emphasizes that willpower alone is insufficient for sustainable weight management. He explains that practical strategies, such as eating nutrient-dense foods and creating enjoyable, realistic lifestyle changes, are essential for long-term success.

Moreover, psychological aspects significantly impact weight loss. The University of Florida's College of Public Health and Health Professions highlights that weight management often involves overcoming deep-seated beliefs and emotional challenges. People struggling with weight can benefit from psychological support and interventions that help them shift their mindset and develop healthier relationships with food and their bodies.

Biological factors also play a crucial role. Metabolic processes, hormone levels, and genetic predispositions can significantly influence one's ability to lose weight. For instance, insulin resistance or thyroid dysfunction can hinder weight loss despite strict adherence to diet and exercise plans. Therefore, addressing these physiological issues through medical evaluation and appropriate interventions is critical.

Additionally, the environment and social factors are pivotal. Access to healthy food options, a supportive community, and structured guidance from professionals like dietitians and health coaches can enhance weight loss efforts. A holistic approach that includes dietary modifications, regular physical activity, stress management, and behavioral changes is more effective than relying solely on willpower.

In summary, weight loss is a multifaceted process that extends beyond mere willpower. It requires a comprehensive strategy that includes practical habits, psychological support, medical interventions, and a supportive environment to achieve and maintain healthy weight management. Understanding and addressing these diverse factors can lead to more sustainable and successful weight loss outcomes.

⎘ External links:

Mayo Clinic News Network — Mayo Clinic Minute: Weight loss and willpower
https://newsnetwork.mayoclinic.org/discussion/mayo-clinic-minute-weight-loss-and-willpower/

UF College of Public Health — It's not all about willpower: A clinical psychologist dispels myths about weight management
https://phhp.ufl.edu/2024/01/31/its-not-all-about-willpower-a-clinical-psychologist-dispels-myths-about-weight-management/

Qilo — The Science of Weight Loss: Understanding Why Weight Loss Isn't Just About Willpower
https://qilo.co/blog/why-weight-loss-isnt-just-about-willpower

Well-Choices Therapy — Weight Loss Myths Debunked
https://well-choices.com/weight-loss-myths-debunked/

Atkins — It's Not Just a Matter of Raw Willpower
https://www.atkins.com/how-it-works/library/articles/its-not-just-a-matter-of-raw-willpower

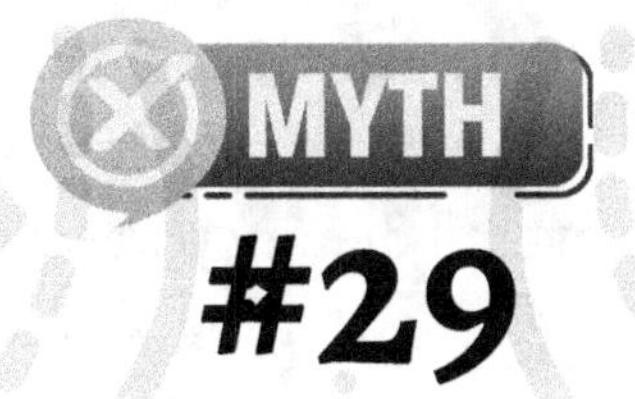

Eating breakfast is essential for weight loss

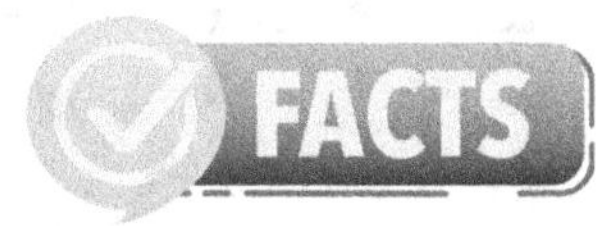

Breakfast is not essential for everyone; individual needs vary.

The idea that eating breakfast is essential for weight loss is a myth that has been debunked by recent research. The necessity of breakfast for weight management varies among individuals and isn't universally essential.

A comprehensive review by The BMJ analyzed multiple randomized controlled trials and found no significant evidence that eating breakfast contributes to weight loss. In fact, some studies indicated a slight weight gain among breakfast eaters compared to those who skipped it. The primary factor in weight loss remains the total caloric intake versus expenditure over the day, rather than the timing of meals.

Moreover, Harvard T.H. Chan School of Public Health highlights that while breakfast can help some people maintain a healthy weight by providing energy and preventing overeating later in the day, it is not a one-size-fits-all solution. Individual metabolic responses and personal habits play a significant role in determining the effectiveness of breakfast in weight management.

WebMD emphasizes that the quality of the diet and mindful eating practices are more crucial than merely eating breakfast. For some, skipping breakfast and following an intermittent fasting regimen might be more effective, provided their overall caloric intake is managed appropriately. The focus should be on a balanced diet rich in nutrients, regardless of whether breakfast is included.

In conclusion, while breakfast can offer benefits such as improved cognitive function and nutrient intake, its role in weight loss is not as significant as previously believed. Individuals should focus on their overall dietary patterns and choose what works best for their bodies and lifestyles. Consulting with a healthcare professional or dietitian can provide personalized guidance tailored to individual needs and goals.

External links:

Harvard Public Health — A healthy breakfast essential to losing weight
https://www.hsph.harvard.edu/news/hsph-in-the-news/a-healthy-breakfast-essential-to-losing-weight/

BMJ — Effect of breakfast on weight and energy intake: systematic review and meta-analysis of randomised controlled trials
https://www.bmj.com/content/364/bmj.l42

Kea Schwarz Functional Nutrition, LLC — The Role of Breakfast in Weight Loss: Myth or Must?
https://www.dietitiankea.com/blog/the-role-of-breakfast-in-weight-loss-myth-or-must

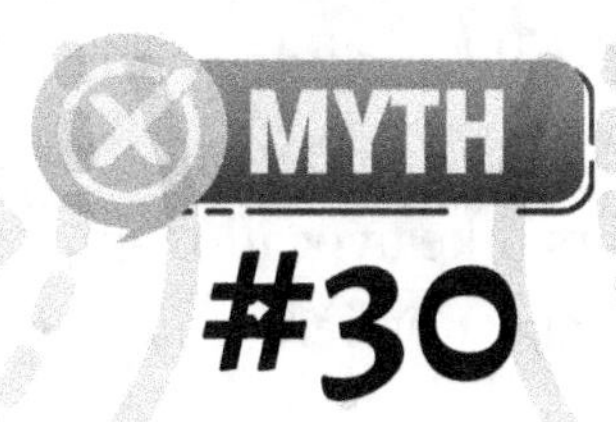

All salads are good for weight loss

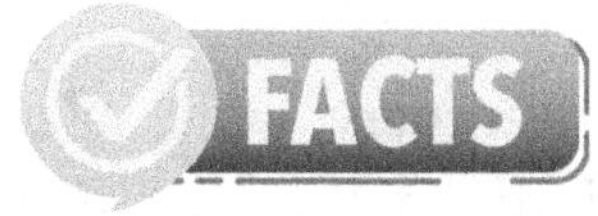

Some salads are high in calories and fat, depending on the ingredients.

The belief that all salads are inherently good for weight loss is a misconception. While salads can be a healthy option, their weight loss benefits depend heavily on the ingredients used. Some salads can be surprisingly high in calories and fat, making them counterproductive for weight loss goals.

A common pitfall is the addition of high-calorie dressings and toppings. Creamy dressings like ranch, blue cheese, and thousand island are often loaded with calories and unhealthy fats. It's better to opt for homemade vinaigrettes or dressings based on olive oil and vinegar, which can be more heart-healthy and lower in calories.

Another issue is the inclusion of fried proteins and processed deli meats. While proteins like chicken, shrimp, and fish are essential for a balanced salad, frying these ingredients can add a significant amount of unhealthy fats and calories. Grilled or baked options are healthier alternatives. Processed meats, such as bacon and deli slices, are also high in calories and sodium, which can derail your weight loss efforts.

Moreover, the type of greens used in salads matters. Iceberg lettuce, while low in calories, lacks the nutritional density of darker leafy greens like spinach, kale, or arugula. These darker greens are richer in vitamins, minerals, and fiber, which are beneficial for overall health and can aid in weight management by keeping you full longer.

For a salad to be truly beneficial for weight loss, it should include a mix of nutrient-dense ingredients. This means plenty of vegetables, lean proteins (such as grilled chicken, beans, or tofu), and healthy fats (like avocados, nuts, and seeds). These components not only provide essential nutrients but also help in maintaining satiety and preventing overeating.

In summary, while salads can be a part of a weight loss diet, it's crucial to be mindful of the ingredients. Avoid high-calorie dressings and toppings, choose nutrient-rich greens, and balance your salad with lean proteins and healthy fats to make it a genuinely weight-friendly meal.

External links:

Anytime Fitness — 10 Common Weight-Loss Myths, Busted
https://www.anytimefitness.com/ccc/ask-a-coach/common-weight-loss-myths-busted/

Livestrong.com — 8 Mistakes to Avoid When Eating Salad for Weight Loss
https://www.livestrong.com/article/13730969-how-to-eat-salad-for-weight-loss/

Verywell Fit — How to Make Salads for Weight Loss
https://www.verywellfit.com/quick-tips-to-make-a-salad-for-weight-loss-3495433

Mcraki Lane — Clean Eating At Home: 30 Make Ahead Salads Under 300 Calories
https://www.merakilane.com/clean-eating-at-home-30-make-ahead-salads-under-300-calories/

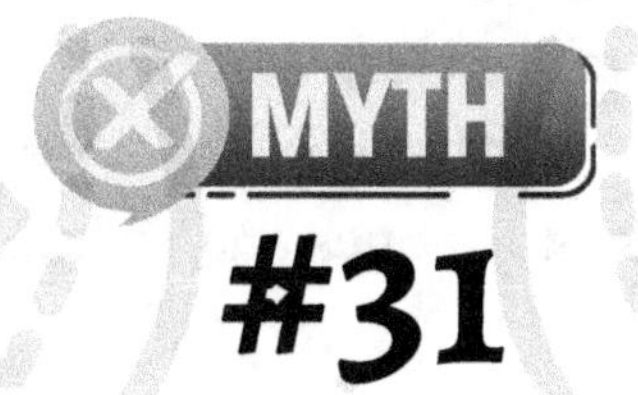

You have to feel hungry to lose weight

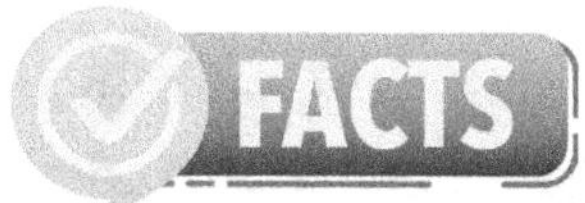

Feeling hungry all the time is not sustainable for weight loss.

The notion that you need to feel hungry to lose weight is a common myth. In reality, constant hunger is not a sustainable or healthy approach to weight loss. Instead, managing hunger effectively through a balanced diet can lead to more successful and long-term weight management.

Feeling hungry all the time can lead to several issues, including overeating and a slowed metabolism. When you consistently restrict calories to the point of significant hunger, your body responds by lowering its metabolic rate to conserve energy. This makes it harder to lose weight and easier to gain it back once you resume normal eating habits.

A better approach is to focus on eating nutrient-dense foods that keep you full and satisfied. High-fiber vegetables, lean proteins, and healthy fats can help control hunger without adding excessive calories. Fiber-rich foods like vegetables and whole grains provide bulk, helping you feel full longer. Proteins, such as chicken, fish, beans, and legumes, are essential for maintaining muscle mass and promoting satiety. Healthy fats, like those found in avocados, nuts, and olive oil, also play a crucial role in feeling full and satisfied.

Another important factor is distinguishing between physical and psychological hunger. Physical hunger is the body's signal that it needs energy, often felt as stomach rumbling or low energy levels. Psychological hunger, on the other hand, can be triggered by emotions, boredom, or habits. Learning to identify and address these triggers can prevent unnecessary eating and support weight loss goals.

Additionally, ensuring adequate sleep is crucial, as lack of sleep can disrupt hunger-regulating hormones, increasing feelings of hunger and cravings. Prioritizing good sleep hygiene can help regulate these hormones and reduce unnecessary hunger.

In summary, sustainable weight loss involves managing hunger through a balanced diet rich in fiber, protein, and healthy fats, rather than enduring constant hunger. This approach not only supports weight loss but also promotes overall health and well-being.

External links:

Diet Doctor — How to Manage Hunger When Trying to Lose Weight
https://www.dietdoctor.com/low-carb/hunger

Livestrong.com — I'm Trying to Lose Weight But Am Always Hungry
https://www.livestrong.com/article/202557-trying-to-lose-weight-but-always-hungry/

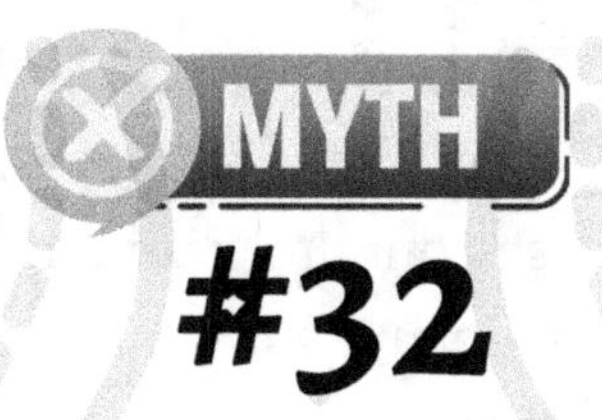

You need to do intense cardio every day to lose weight

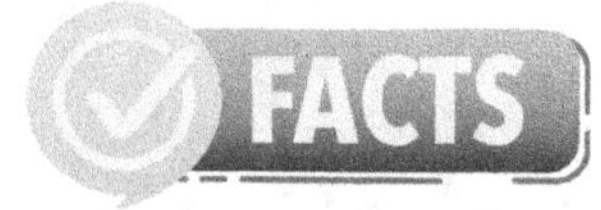

Cardio is important, but strength training and rest are also crucial.

The belief that intense cardio every day is necessary for weight loss is a myth. While cardio is an important component of a fitness routine, incorporating strength training and allowing for rest are equally crucial for effective and sustainable weight loss.

Cardio exercises, such as running, cycling, or high-intensity interval training (HIIT), are excellent for burning calories and improving cardiovascular health. However, focusing solely on cardio can lead to diminishing returns and potential burnout. It's essential to combine cardio with strength training to maximize the benefits. Strength training builds muscle mass, which increases the body's resting metabolic rate, meaning you burn more calories even when not exercising.

Strength training should not be overlooked in a weight loss regimen. It not only helps in building muscle but also supports joint health, improves balance, and enhances overall strength. Incorporating exercises like weight lifting, resistance band workouts, or bodyweight exercises can significantly contribute to your fitness goals.

Moreover, rest and recovery are vital. Muscles need time to repair and grow after workouts. Overtraining can lead to injuries, fatigue, and decreased performance. Ensuring you have rest days or engage in active recovery, such as light stretching or yoga, can help maintain a balanced and effective workout routine.

For those looking to optimize their exercise regimen, a balanced approach is recommended. This could include moderate-intensity cardio sessions several times a week, combined with strength training exercises on alternate days. High-intensity interval training (HIIT) can also be beneficial, as it combines both cardio and strength elements and can be done in shorter, more efficient sessions.

In conclusion, while cardio is important for weight loss, integrating strength training and allowing for adequate rest are essential for a well-rounded and sustainable fitness program. This approach not only helps in losing weight but also in maintaining overall health and fitness.

⬈ External links:

Mayo Clinic Health System — Debunking the top 10 workout myths
https://www.mayoclinichealthsystem.org/hometown-health/speaking-of-health/top-10-workout-myths

Verywell Fit — Cardio and Strength Training: Why You Should Do Both
https://www.verywellfit.com/cardio-and-weight-training-and-fat-loss-3498325

Verywell Fit — Cardio Workouts: What You Need to Know
https://www.verywellfit.com/everything-you-need-to-know-about-cardio-1229553

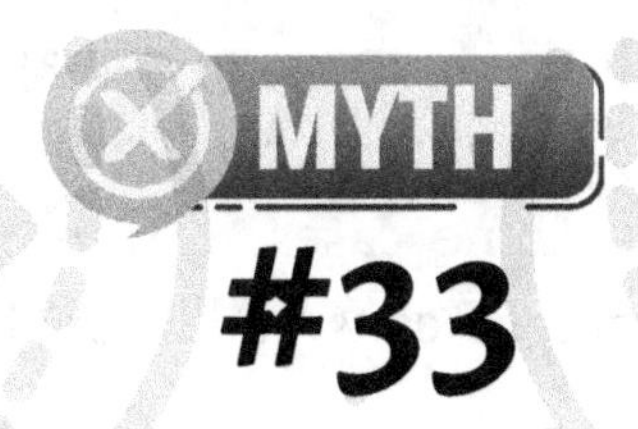

Low-carb diets are the best way to lose weight

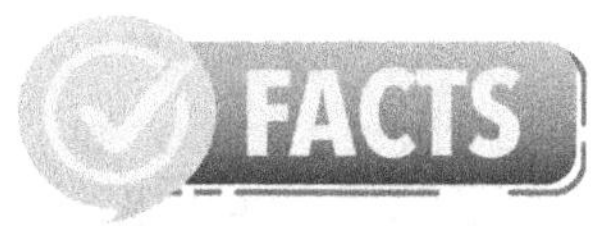

Low-carb diets work for some, but not everyone.

The idea that low-carb diets are the best way to lose weight is a common misconception. While low-carb diets can be effective for some people, they are not universally the best approach for everyone. The success of any diet largely depends on individual preferences, metabolic responses, and lifestyle sustainability.

Low-carb diets, which limit foods high in carbohydrates like bread, pasta, and certain fruits, can lead to short-term weight loss primarily due to water weight reduction and decreased calorie intake. These diets often emphasize protein and fat, which can help increase feelings of fullness and reduce overall calorie consumption. However, the long-term benefits of low-carb diets are not significantly greater than those of other dietary approaches.

One major drawback of low-carb diets is their sustainability. Many people find it challenging to adhere to such restrictive eating patterns over the long term. This can lead to a cycle of losing and regaining weight, which is not ideal for long-term health and weight management.

Additionally, a balanced diet that includes a variety of nutrients from all food groups is essential for overall health. Complex carbohydrates, such as whole grains, fruits, and vegetables, provide essential vitamins, minerals, and fiber that support digestive health, stabilize blood sugar levels, and reduce the risk of chronic diseases like heart disease and type 2 diabetes.

Moreover, individual responses to low-carb diets can vary. Some people may experience side effects like constipation, headaches, and muscle cramps due to the sudden reduction in carbohydrate intake. In some cases, extreme carbohydrate restriction can lead to ketosis, which might cause additional side effects like bad breath and fatigue.

In summary, while low-carb diets can be an effective weight loss strategy for some, they are not the best or most sustainable approach for everyone. A balanced diet that includes a moderate amount of carbohydrates, combined with regular physical activity, is generally recommended for long-term weight management and overall health.

⬈ External links:

Mayo Clinic — Low-carb diet: Can it help you lose weight?
https://www.mayoclinic.org/healthy-lifestyle/weight-loss/in-depth/low-carb-diet/art-20045831

My Vanderbilt Health — Do Carbs Make You Gain Weight? 4 Myths Debunked by Dietitian
https://my.vanderbilthealth.com/debunking-4-common-carb-myths/

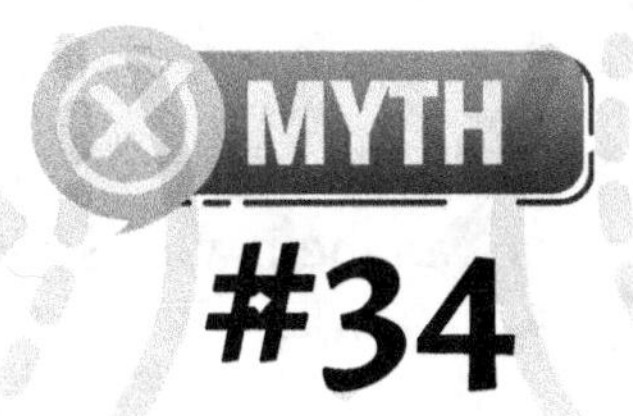

You can't eat out and still lose weight

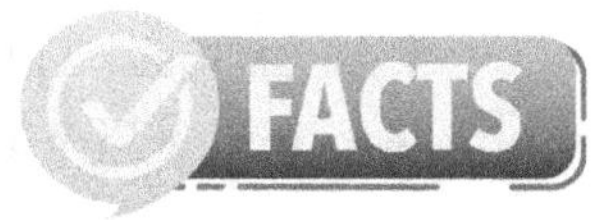

You can make healthy choices when eating out to support weight loss.

The myth that you can't eat out and still lose weight is simply not true. With mindful choices and a bit of preparation, dining out can fit into a healthy weight loss plan.

Firstly, it's important to focus on balance and moderation rather than restriction. When dining out, opt for dishes that include lean proteins, vegetables, and whole grains. For instance, choosing grilled chicken over fried options, requesting sauces and dressings on the side, and prioritizing steamed vegetables can significantly reduce calorie intake without sacrificing enjoyment.

Portion control is another key factor. Restaurants often serve larger portions than necessary, which can lead to overeating. Consider splitting a meal with a friend, ordering an appetizer as your main dish, or immediately boxing half of your entrée to take home. This helps manage portions and prevents overconsumption.

Additionally, paying attention to how the food is prepared can make a big difference. Opt for baked, grilled, or steamed dishes rather than those that are fried or sautéed in heavy oils and butter. For example, instead of deep-fried items, go for grilled fish or chicken, which are lower in unhealthy fats and calories.

Beverage choices also matter. Sugary drinks, including sodas and sweetened teas, can add a significant number of empty calories to your meal. Choosing water, unsweetened tea, or other low-calorie beverages can help you stay within your calorie goals while still enjoying your dining experience.

Lastly, practicing mindful eating can enhance the dining experience and support weight loss. Taking the time to savor each bite, eating slowly, and paying attention to hunger and fullness cues can prevent overeating and make the meal more satisfying.

By making informed choices and being mindful of portions and preparation methods, you can enjoy eating out while still achieving your weight loss goals. It's all about balance, moderation, and making healthier choices that align with your lifestyle.

External links:

WW — 10 Weight Loss Myths | Starvation Mode + More
https://www.weightwatchers.com/us/blog/weight-loss/top-weight-loss-myths

Mayo Clinic Diet — Eat what you love and still lose weight
https://diet.mayoclinic.org/us/blog/2022/eat-what-you-love-and-still-lose-weight/

Eat This Not That — 20 Weight Loss Myths—Busted
https://www.eatthis.com/weight-loss-myths/

NIDDK — Some Myths about Nutrition & Physical Activity
https://www.niddk.nih.gov/health-information/weight-management/myths-nutrition-physical-activity

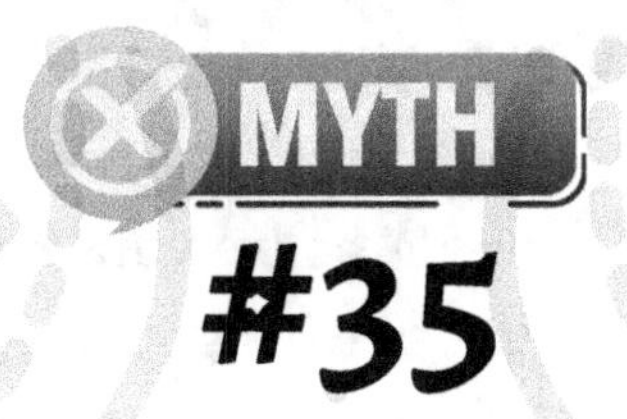

Weight loss is linear and should happen steadily

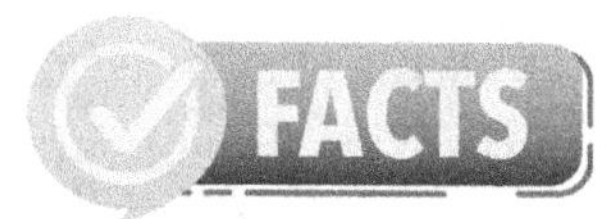

Weight loss can be unpredictable and varies from person to person.

The belief that weight loss is linear and should happen steadily is a common myth. In reality, weight loss can be unpredictable and varies significantly from person to person due to various factors including biological, hormonal, and lifestyle influences.

Initially, weight loss might occur rapidly due to the loss of water weight and glycogen stores. However, as you continue on your weight loss journey, the rate of weight loss can slow down and even plateau. This is because the body adapts to the changes in diet and exercise, and metabolic rates may decrease as muscle mass is lost along with fat.

Daily weight fluctuations are also normal and can be influenced by factors such as water retention, menstrual cycles, and the type and timing of food consumed. This means that day-to-day changes on the scale do not necessarily reflect actual fat loss or gain.

Moreover, individual differences in metabolism, genetics, and hormonal balance play a significant role in how people lose weight. For instance, some individuals may lose weight more quickly at the beginning and then experience periods of little to no weight loss, which can be frustrating but is entirely normal.

To better track progress, it's helpful to look beyond the scale. Measuring body composition, such as changes in body measurements or how clothes fit, can provide a more accurate picture of progress. Tools like 3D body scans or regular measurements of waist, hips, and other areas can offer insights into fat loss and muscle gain.

Ultimately, sustainable weight loss involves patience and persistence. It's important to focus on overall health improvements, such as better energy levels, improved fitness, and healthier eating habits, rather than just the number on the scale. Adopting a balanced approach to diet and exercise, and setting realistic expectations, can help manage the frustrations that come with the non-linear nature of weight loss.

External links:

Calibrate — Weight Loss Myths: 6 Biggest Weight Loss Myths, Busted
https://www.joincalibrate.com/resources/weight-loss-myths

ZOZOFIT — Why Weight Loss Is Not Linear and How To Track Your Progress
https://zozofit.com/blogs/news/why-weight-loss-is-not-linear-and-how-to-track-your-progress

Eat This Not That — 20 Weight Loss Myths—Busted!
https://www.eatthis.com/weight-loss-myths/

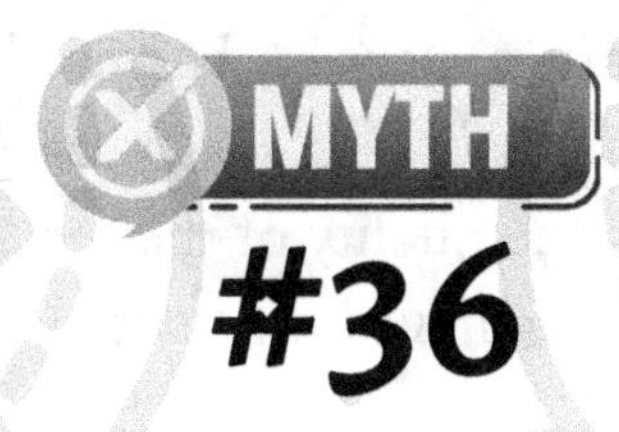

All sugar is bad for weight loss

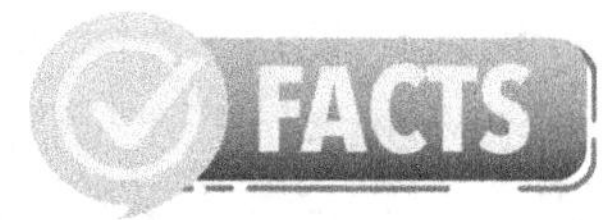

Natural sugars can be part of a healthy diet.

The idea that all sugar is bad for weight loss is a myth. In reality, natural sugars, such as those found in fruits and dairy products, can be part of a healthy diet and even support weight loss when consumed in moderation.

Natural sugars in fruits (fructose) and dairy (lactose) come packaged with essential nutrients like fiber, vitamins, and minerals. For example, fruits provide fiber which helps in digestion and promotes a feeling of fullness, reducing overall calorie intake. Dairy products like milk and unsweetened yogurt offer protein and calcium, which are crucial for maintaining muscle mass and bone health.

The primary concern with sugar intake is often the consumption of added sugars, which are found in processed foods and sugary beverages. These added sugars contribute extra calories without any nutritional benefits, leading to weight gain and other health issues if consumed in excess. Therefore, it is important to limit foods with added sugars such as sweets, sugary drinks, and processed snacks.

While it might seem beneficial to replace sugar with low- or no-calorie sweeteners, these alternatives can sometimes lead to increased cravings for sweet foods and may not provide the expected weight loss benefits. It's better to focus on reducing overall sugar intake and opting for natural sources of sweetness from whole foods.

Additionally, it is crucial to consider the overall dietary pattern. A balanced diet rich in whole, minimally processed foods, including fruits and dairy, can support weight loss and overall health. By focusing on the quality of the food and maintaining a calorie deficit, weight loss can be achieved without the need to eliminate natural sugars from the diet.

In summary, natural sugars from fruits and dairy can be part of a healthy diet and support weight loss, whereas added sugars should be limited. It's about finding a balance and making informed choices that contribute to long-term health and well-being.

External links:

Livestrong.com — 5 Myths About Sugar That Could Prevent You From Losing Weight
https://www.livestrong.com/article/13776220-myths-about-sugar-and-weight-loss/

HealthBehavSci — Debunking 10 Common Nutrition Myths
https://habs.uq.edu.au/blog/2023/10/debunking-10-common-nutrition-myths

EverydayHealth.com — Which Sugars Are Good for You — and Which Ones to Avoid
https://www.everydayhealth.com/diet-and-nutrition/diet/which-sugars-are-good-you-which-ones-avoid/

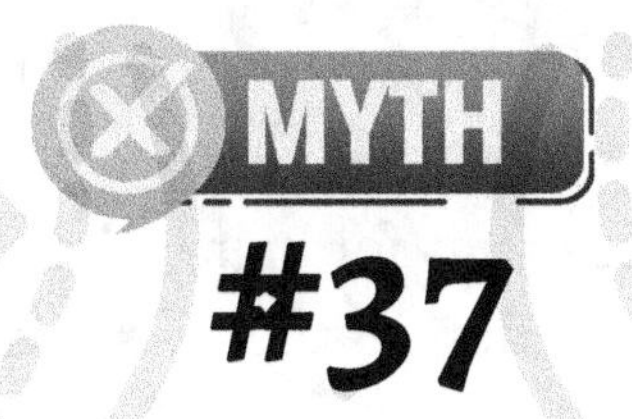

Drinking coffee leads to weight gain

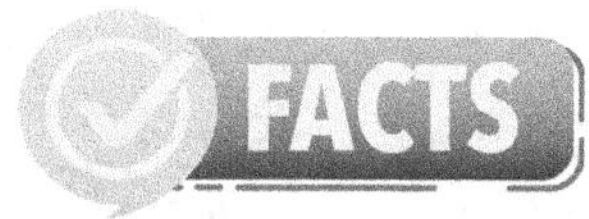

Coffee can aid metabolism when consumed in moderation.

The belief that drinking coffee leads to weight gain is a myth. In fact, when consumed in moderation, coffee can aid metabolism and support weight loss efforts.

Coffee contains caffeine, a natural stimulant that can boost metabolic rate by 3-11%, depending on the amount consumed. This increase in metabolism helps the body burn more calories, even at rest. Additionally, caffeine can enhance the breakdown of fat cells, making them available as a source of energy during physical activities.

Moreover, coffee can act as an appetite suppressant, reducing feelings of hunger and helping to control calorie intake. Drinking black coffee before meals can help you feel fuller and potentially eat less, contributing to a calorie deficit necessary for weight loss.

However, it's important to consider how coffee is consumed. Adding high-calorie ingredients such as sugar, flavored syrups, whipped cream, and full-fat milk can turn a low-calorie beverage into a calorie-laden treat, which can undermine weight loss efforts. For instance, a few tablespoons of flavored creamer can add significant calories and sugars, leading to potential weight gain if consumed regularly.

Sleep quality is another factor to consider. Drinking coffee late in the day can disrupt sleep patterns, leading to poor sleep quality and subsequent weight gain, as poor sleep is linked to increased hunger and cravings for high-calorie foods. Therefore, it's advisable to limit coffee consumption to the morning and early afternoon to avoid sleep disruptions.

In summary, coffee, particularly black coffee, can support weight loss by boosting metabolism and suppressing appetite. However, it's crucial to avoid high-calorie additives and be mindful of consumption times to prevent negative impacts on sleep. A balanced approach, combining moderate coffee intake with a healthy diet and regular exercise, is key to leveraging coffee's benefits for weight management.

External links:

PreventiveMedDaily — Debunking Common Myths About Coffee and Weight Loss: Separating Fact from Fiction
https://www.preventivemedicinedaily.com/healthy-living/weight-loss/debunking-common-myths-about-coffee-and-weight-loss-separating-fact-from-fiction/

Buoy Health — Does Caffeine Cause Weight Gain or Weight Loss? Experts Weigh In
https://www.buoyhealth.com/weight-management/caffeine-and-weight-gain

Gateway Region YMCA — But First, Coffee: Can Caffeine Impact Your Workout?
https://gwrymca.org/blog/effects-of-caffeine-on-exercise

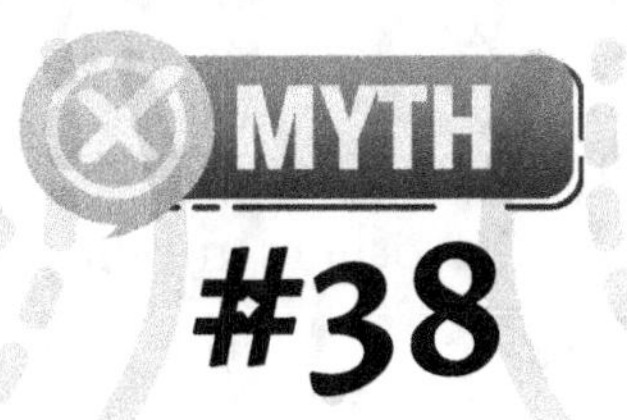

You must follow the same diet as your friend to lose weight

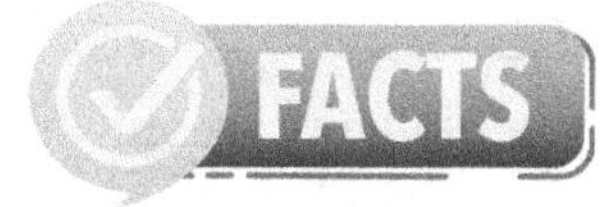

Individual responses to diets vary; personalized approaches work best.

The notion that you must follow the same diet as your friend to lose weight is a myth. Individual responses to diets vary significantly, and a personalized approach is often more effective for achieving and maintaining weight loss.

One major factor in this variability is metabolic rate. Research shows that people have different basal metabolic rates (BMR), which means they burn calories at different rates even while at rest. This can influence how effectively a particular diet works for an individual. For instance, a study found that competitors on "The Biggest Loser" who maintained their weight loss had significantly lower BMRs than those who regained weight, highlighting the need for personalized diet plans that consider metabolic differences.

Moreover, genetics and gut microbiota play crucial roles in how our bodies respond to different diets. Genetic variations can affect how efficiently we process and store energy from food. Similarly, the composition of gut bacteria, which helps in nutrient absorption and metabolism, varies from person to person. This suggests that some individuals may require different dietary adjustments to achieve optimal weight loss.

A personalized diet approach also considers individual preferences, lifestyle, and any medical conditions. The Mayo Clinic emphasizes that successful weight loss requires a sustainable plan that includes foods you enjoy and can easily incorporate into your lifestyle. A diet that is too restrictive or does not align with your tastes is likely to fail in the long term.

Additionally, different diets have varying impacts on satiety and hunger hormones, which can affect adherence and success. For example, some people might feel more satisfied on a higher protein diet, while others might do better with more complex carbohydrates and fiber.

In conclusion, a personalized approach to dieting, tailored to an individual's metabolic rate, genetic makeup, gut microbiota, and personal preferences, is more likely to result in sustainable weight loss compared to following a friend's diet plan. It's essential to find a balanced and flexible diet that fits your unique needs and lifestyle.

⬀ External links:

Mayo Clinic — Weight loss: 6 strategies for success
https://www.mayoclinic.org/healthy-lifestyle/weight-loss/in-depth/weight-loss/art-20047752

Mayo Clinic — Weight loss: Choosing a diet that's right for you
https://www.mayoclinic.org/healthy-lifestyle/weight-loss/in-depth/weight-loss/art-20048466

Today's Dietitian — Weight Loss Resistance — Myth or Harsh Reality?
https://www.todaysdietitian.com/newarchives/0716p32.shtml

More protein always means more weight loss

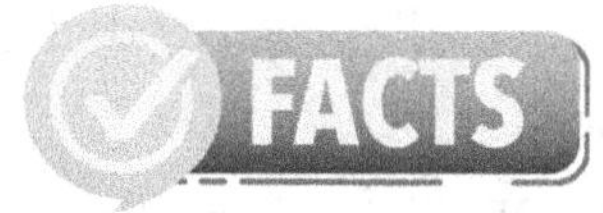

Protein is important, but balance with other nutrients is essential.

The belief that consuming more protein always leads to more weight loss is a common myth. While protein is an important component of a healthy diet and can support weight loss efforts, balance with other nutrients is essential for optimal health and sustainable weight loss.

Protein plays a crucial role in maintaining muscle mass, especially during weight loss, as it helps preserve lean body mass while promoting fat loss. It also has a high thermic effect, meaning the body burns more calories digesting protein compared to carbohydrates and fats. This can contribute to a slight increase in metabolism and help with satiety, making you feel fuller for longer and potentially reducing overall calorie intake.

However, an excessively high-protein diet is not without its downsides. Consuming more protein than the body needs does not necessarily lead to more muscle gain or weight loss. Instead, the excess protein can be converted to glucose and potentially stored as fat. Additionally, high-protein diets can be hard on the kidneys, especially for those with preexisting kidney conditions, and may lead to nutrient imbalances if other essential nutrients are neglected.

Balancing protein intake with carbohydrates and fats is vital. Carbohydrates are the body's primary energy source, and they are essential for fueling physical activity and brain function. Fats are important for hormone production, brain health, and absorbing fat-soluble vitamins. A balanced diet that includes a variety of protein sources—both animal and plant-based—alongside fruits, vegetables, whole grains, and healthy fats is recommended for overall health and effective weight management.

In conclusion, while protein is a key nutrient for weight loss, it should be consumed as part of a balanced diet that includes all essential nutrients. Personalized dietary approaches, considering individual health needs and preferences, are more effective for sustainable weight loss and overall well-being.

External links:

MyFitnessPal Blog — The Essential Guide to Protein for Optimal Health
https://blog.myfitnesspal.com/essential-guide-to-protein/

The Balanced Nutritionist — Facts About Protein From a Registered Dietitian
https://thebalancednutritionist.com/facts-about-protein/

Cleveland Clinic — How Much Protein To Eat To Lose Weight
https://health.clevelandclinic.org/how-much-protein-to-eat-to-lose-weight

Verywell Fit — How Much Protein Should I Eat to Lose Weight?
https://www.verywellfit.com/how-much-protein-is-best-for-weight-loss-3495783

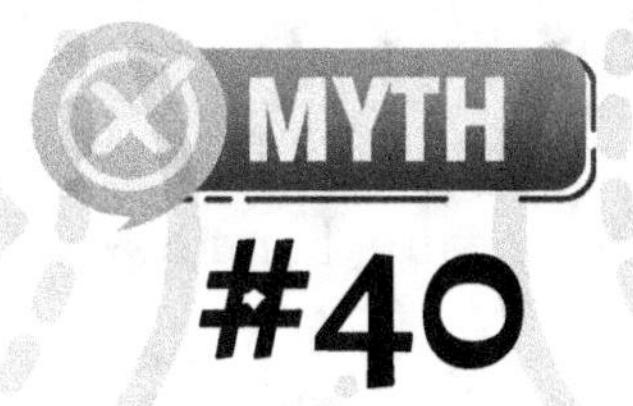

Healthy food is always more expensive

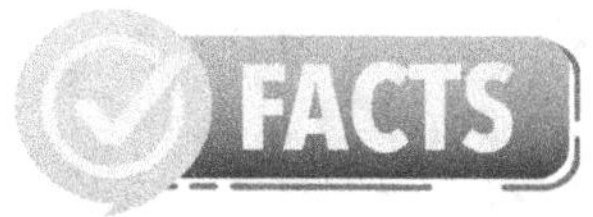

Healthy eating can be affordable with proper planning.

The idea that healthy food is always more expensive is a common myth. In reality, healthy eating can be affordable with proper planning and smart shopping strategies.

First, planning meals and snacks around sales and seasonal produce can significantly reduce costs. Seasonal fruits and vegetables are often cheaper and fresher. Additionally, creating a shopping list and sticking to it helps avoid impulse buys and ensures you purchase only what you need.

Buying in bulk is another effective strategy. Staple items such as whole grains, beans, nuts, and seeds can be purchased in larger quantities at a lower cost per unit. This approach not only saves money but also reduces the frequency of shopping trips.

Another way to eat healthily on a budget is to opt for store brands over name brands. Many generic or store-brand products contain the same ingredients as their branded counterparts but are significantly cheaper due to lower marketing and packaging costs.

Frozen and canned fruits and vegetables are also excellent, cost-effective alternatives to fresh produce. These options are often just as nutritious as fresh ones and have a longer shelf life, which helps reduce food waste. It's important to choose options without added sugars or salt to maintain nutritional quality.

A study by the Harvard School of Public Health found that the healthiest diets cost only about $1.50 more per day than the least healthy diets. This slight increase in daily cost can be offset by the long-term health benefits and reduced healthcare costs associated with a healthy diet.

In conclusion, eating healthy doesn't have to break the bank. With thoughtful planning, bulk buying, choosing store brands, and using frozen and canned produce, it's entirely possible to maintain a nutritious diet on a budget.

External links:

Tufts Nutrition Letter — Mythbusting: The Cost of Healthy Eating
https://www.nutritionletter.tufts.edu/special-reports/mythbusting-the-cost-of-healthy-eating/

Mayo Clinic Health System — 10 common nutrition myths debunked
https://www.mayoclinichealthsystem.org/hometown-health/speaking-of-health/10-nutrition-myths-debunked

The Nutrition Source — Strategies for Eating Well on a Budget
https://nutritionsource.hsph.harvard.edu/strategies-nutrition-budget/

Harvard Public Health — Eating healthy vs. unhealthy diet costs about $1.50 more per day
https://www.hsph.harvard.edu/news/press-releases/healthy-vs-unhealthy-diet-costs-1-50-more/

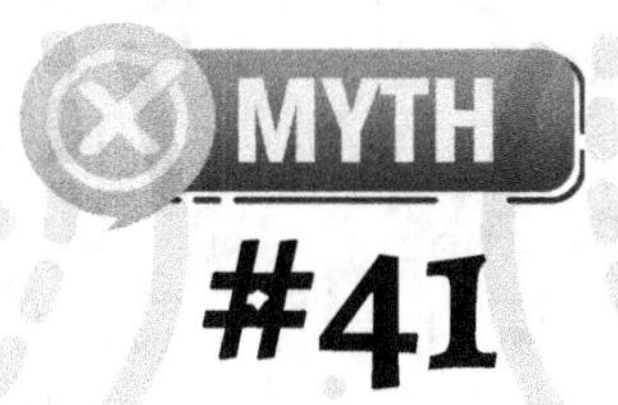

Drinking coffee leads to weight gain

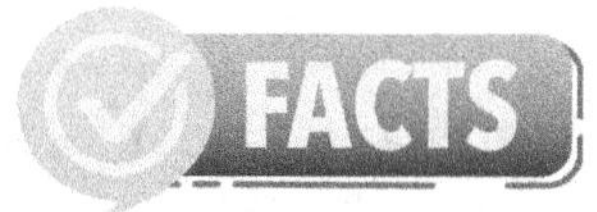

Plain coffee has minimal calories and can even boost metabolism. It's the added sugars and creams that can lead to weight gain.

Many people believe that drinking coffee leads to weight gain, but this is largely a myth. Plain coffee has minimal calories and can actually boost metabolism, aiding in weight management. It's the added sugars, creamers, and other high-calorie ingredients that can lead to weight gain.

Black coffee is virtually calorie-free, with an 8-ounce cup containing only about five calories. This makes it an excellent choice for those looking to maintain or lose weight. Coffee can also increase your metabolic rate, helping you burn more calories at rest. Drinking coffee before exercise has been shown to improve performance, which can further support weight loss efforts.

However, the way you consume your coffee matters significantly. Adding sugar, whipped cream, flavored syrups, and high-fat milk or cream can turn a low-calorie beverage into a high-calorie indulgence. These additions contribute to increased calorie intake and can negate the potential weight management benefits of coffee.

Another factor to consider is the timing of coffee consumption. Drinking coffee late in the day can interfere with sleep, and poor sleep is associated with weight gain. Lack of sleep can disrupt hormones that regulate hunger, leading to increased cravings and calorie intake.

To enjoy coffee without the risk of weight gain, consider drinking it black or with minimal low-calorie additions. Opt for unsweetened plant-based milks if you prefer a milk alternative, and gradually reduce the amount of sugar and sweeteners you use. Making coffee at home can also help control the ingredients and portion sizes, reducing the temptation of high-calorie coffee shop beverages.

In summary, plain coffee is a low-calorie beverage that can boost metabolism and support weight management. The key is to avoid high-calorie additions and consume coffee in a way that doesn't disrupt your sleep.

External links:

mindbodygreen — 5 Sneaky Reasons Coffee Can Cause Weight Gain & What To Do
https://www.mindbodygreen.com/articles/drinking-caffeine-can-cause-weight-gain-heres-how

DrBrahma — Coffee and Weight Gain: Understanding the Facts and Myths Behind Your Morning Cup
https://www.drbrahma.com/coffee-and-weight-gain-facts-you-must-know/

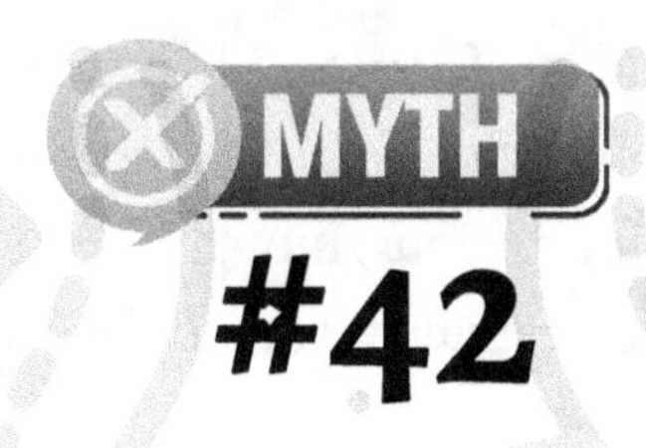

You must follow the same diet as your friends or family to lose weight

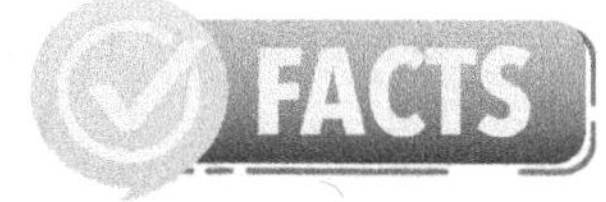

Everyone's body is different. The best diet for weight loss is one that suits your individual needs and preferences.

The notion that you must follow the same diet as your friend to lose weight is a myth. Individual responses to diets vary significantly, and a personalized approach is often more effective for achieving and maintaining weight loss.

One major factor in this variability is metabolic rate. Research shows that people have different basal metabolic rates (BMR), which means they burn calories at different rates even while at rest. This can influence how effectively a particular diet works for an individual. For instance, a study found that competitors on "The Biggest Loser" who maintained their weight loss had significantly lower BMRs than those who regained weight, highlighting the need for personalized diet plans that consider metabolic differences.

Moreover, genetics and gut microbiota play crucial roles in how our bodies respond to different diets. Genetic variations can affect how efficiently we process and store energy from food. Similarly, the composition of gut bacteria, which helps in nutrient absorption and metabolism, varies from person to person. This suggests that some individuals may require different dietary adjustments to achieve optimal weight loss.

A personalized diet approach also considers individual preferences, lifestyle, and any medical conditions. The Mayo Clinic emphasizes that successful weight loss requires a sustainable plan that includes foods you enjoy and can easily incorporate into your lifestyle. A diet that is too restrictive or does not align with your tastes is likely to fail in the long term.

Additionally, different diets have varying impacts on satiety and hunger hormones, which can affect adherence and success. For example, some people might feel more satisfied on a higher protein diet, while others might do better with more complex carbohydrates and fiber.

In conclusion, a personalized approach to dieting, tailored to an individual's metabolic rate, genetic makeup, gut microbiota, and personal preferences, is more likely to result in sustainable weight loss compared to following a friend's diet plan. It's essential to find a balanced and flexible diet that fits your unique needs and lifestyle.

⤴ External links:

Mayo Clinic — Weight loss: 6 strategies for success
https://www.mayoclinic.org/healthy-lifestyle/weight-loss/in-depth/weight-loss/art-20047752

Mayo Clinic — Weight loss: Choosing a diet that's right for you
https://www.mayoclinic.org/healthy-lifestyle/weight-loss/in-depth/weight-loss/art-20048466

Today's Dietitian — Weight Loss Resistance — Myth or Harsh Reality?
https://www.todaysdietitian.com/newarchives/0716p32.shtml

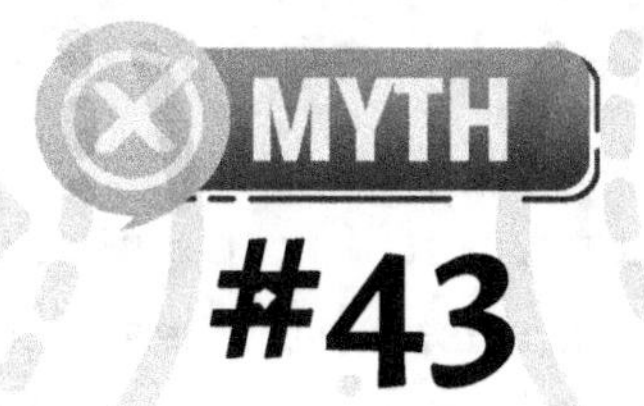

More protein always means more weight loss

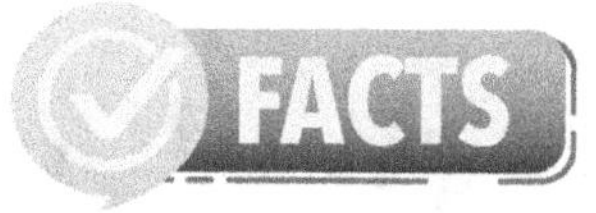

Protein is important, but balance with other nutrients is essential.

The belief that consuming more protein always leads to more weight loss is a common myth. While protein is an important component of a healthy diet and can support weight loss efforts, balance with other nutrients is essential for optimal health and sustainable weight loss.

Protein plays a crucial role in maintaining muscle mass, especially during weight loss, as it helps preserve lean body mass while promoting fat loss. It also has a high thermic effect, meaning the body burns more calories digesting protein compared to carbohydrates and fats. This can contribute to a slight increase in metabolism and help with satiety, making you feel fuller for longer and potentially reducing overall calorie intake.

However, an excessively high-protein diet is not without its downsides. Consuming more protein than the body needs does not necessarily lead to more muscle gain or weight loss. Instead, the excess protein can be converted to glucose and potentially stored as fat. Additionally, high-protein diets can be hard on the kidneys, especially for those with preexisting kidney conditions, and may lead to nutrient imbalances if other essential nutrients are neglected.

Balancing protein intake with carbohydrates and fats is vital. Carbohydrates are the body's primary energy source, and they are essential for fueling physical activity and brain function. Fats are important for hormone production, brain health, and absorbing fat-soluble vitamins. A balanced diet that includes a variety of protein sources—both animal and plant-based—alongside fruits, vegetables, whole grains, and healthy fats is recommended for overall health and effective weight management.

In conclusion, while protein is a key nutrient for weight loss, it should be consumed as part of a balanced diet that includes all essential nutrients. Personalized dietary approaches, considering individual health needs and preferences, are more effective for sustainable weight loss and overall well-being.

⤴ External links:

MyFitnessPal Blog — The Essential Guide to Protein for Optimal Health
https://blog.myfitnesspal.com/essential-guide-to-protein/

The Balanced Nutritionist — Facts About Protein From a Registered Dietitian
https://thebalancednutritionist.com/facts-about-protein/

Cleveland Clinic — How Much Protein To Eat To Lose Weight
https://health.clevelandclinic.org/how-much-protein-to-eat-to-lose-weight

Verywell Fit — How Much Protein Should I Eat to Lose Weight?
https://www.verywellfit.com/how-much-protein-is-best-for-weight-loss-3495783

Healthy food is always more expensive

Healthy eating can be affordable with proper planning.

The idea that healthy food is always more expensive is a common myth. In reality, healthy eating can be affordable with proper planning and smart shopping strategies.

First, planning meals and snacks around sales and seasonal produce can significantly reduce costs. Seasonal fruits and vegetables are often cheaper and fresher. Additionally, creating a shopping list and sticking to it helps avoid impulse buys and ensures you purchase only what you need.

Buying in bulk is another effective strategy. Staple items such as whole grains, beans, nuts, and seeds can be purchased in larger quantities at a lower cost per unit. This approach not only saves money but also reduces the frequency of shopping trips.

Another way to eat healthily on a budget is to opt for store brands over name brands. Many generic or store-brand products contain the same ingredients as their branded counterparts but are significantly cheaper due to lower marketing and packaging costs.

Frozen and canned fruits and vegetables are also excellent, cost-effective alternatives to fresh produce. These options are often just as nutritious as fresh ones and have a longer shelf life, which helps reduce food waste. It's important to choose options without added sugars or salt to maintain nutritional quality.

A study by the Harvard School of Public Health found that the healthiest diets cost only about $1.50 more per day than the least healthy diets. This slight increase in daily cost can be offset by the long-term health benefits and reduced healthcare costs associated with a healthy diet.

In conclusion, eating healthy doesn't have to break the bank. With thoughtful planning, bulk buying, choosing store brands, and using frozen and canned produce, it's entirely possible to maintain a nutritious diet on a budget.

External links:

Mayo Clinic Health System — 10 common nutrition myths debunked
https://www.mayoclinichealthsystem.org/hometown-health/speaking-of-health/10-nutrition-myths-debunked

The Nutrition Source — Strategies for Eating Well on a Budget
https://nutritionsource.hsph.harvard.edu/strategies-nutrition-budget/

Harvard School of Public Health — Eating healthy vs. unhealthy diet costs about $1.50 more per day
https://www.hsph.harvard.edu/news/press-releases/healthy-vs-unhealthy-diet-costs-1-50-more/

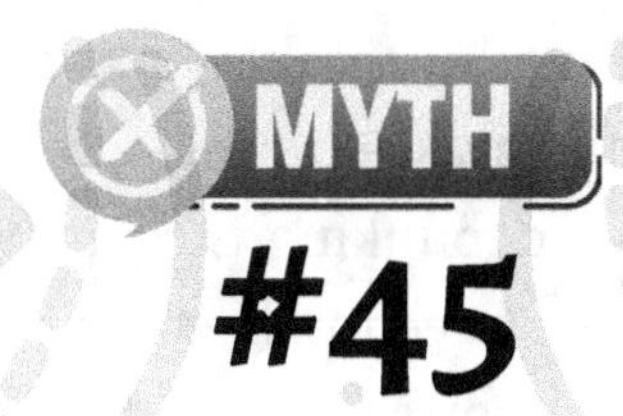

You can't gain muscle while losing fat

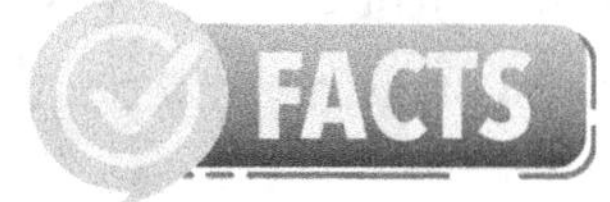

With the right balance of nutrition and exercise, it's possible to gain muscle and lose fat simultaneously.

The belief that you can't gain muscle while losing fat is a persistent myth. However, with the right balance of nutrition and exercise, achieving both simultaneously is indeed possible. This concept is known as body recomposition.

The crux of the myth is rooted in the traditional understanding that muscle gain requires a caloric surplus, while fat loss necessitates a caloric deficit. While it seems contradictory, research and practical evidence suggest that these processes can coexist under specific conditions.

Firstly, nutrition plays a crucial role. High protein intake is essential for preserving muscle mass during a caloric deficit. Consuming between 1 to 1.2 grams of protein per pound of body weight helps maintain muscle while promoting fat loss. Additionally, timing meals around workouts and slightly increasing calorie intake on training days can optimize muscle gain without hindering fat loss.

Exercise is equally important. Resistance training, such as weightlifting, stimulates muscle growth even in a caloric deficit. Incorporating compound movements like squats, deadlifts, and bench presses can maximize muscle hypertrophy and metabolic rate, aiding in fat loss. Cardiovascular exercise also supports fat loss but should be balanced to avoid excessive muscle breakdown.

Scientific studies back these approaches. For example, a study highlighted by McMaster University found that individuals could gain muscle and lose fat through structured exercise and nutritional strategies, debunking the myth that these goals are mutually exclusive. Furthermore, anecdotal evidence from fitness professionals and bodybuilders supports this claim, demonstrating practical success in achieving body recomposition.

In conclusion, while the process of gaining muscle and losing fat simultaneously is slower than focusing on one goal at a time, it is achievable. A strategic approach combining high protein intake, meal timing, resistance training, and appropriate cardiovascular exercise can lead to successful body recomposition.

External links:

BarBend — How To Lose Fat and Gain Muscle, According to Science
https://barbend.com/how-to-lose-fat-and-gain-muscle-according-to-science/

ScienceDaily — Losing fat while gaining muscle: Scientists close in on 'holy grail' of diet and exercise
https://www.sciencedaily.com/releases/2016/01/160127132741.htm

Bodybuilding.com — Build Muscle And Lose Fat Simultaneously: Yes, It Is Possible!
https://www.bodybuilding.com/content/build-muscle-and-lose-fat-simultaneously-yes-it-is-possible.html

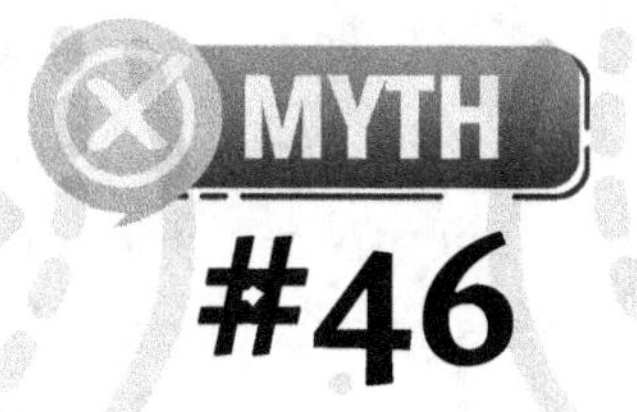

Organic foods always lead to weight loss

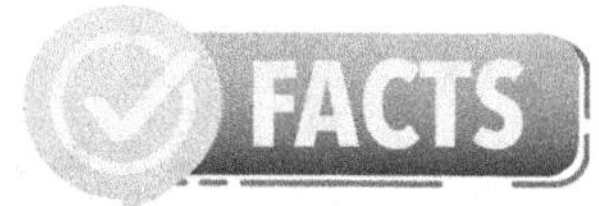

Organic foods can still be high in calories. Weight loss depends on overall diet quality and calorie balance.

The notion that organic foods inherently lead to weight loss is a common myth. While organic foods are often perceived as healthier, they are not necessarily lower in calories. Weight loss fundamentally depends on the balance between the calories consumed and the calories burned, rather than simply the type of food ingested.

Organic foods can still be high in calories. For example, organic cookies or snacks might be free from synthetic pesticides and fertilizers, but they still contain sugars and fats, which contribute to their calorie content. Thus, consuming large quantities of organic foods can still lead to weight gain if calorie intake exceeds what your body needs.

Moreover, the term "organic" refers to how food is produced. Organic farming emphasizes the use of natural substances and processes, avoiding synthetic pesticides and fertilizers. While this can mean fewer chemical residues, it doesn't inherently make the food lower in calories or more conducive to weight loss.

For effective weight management, it is crucial to focus on overall diet quality and maintaining a calorie deficit. Incorporating a variety of nutrient-dense foods, whether organic or not, and balancing macronutrients can support weight loss goals. Regular physical activity also plays a significant role in burning calories and promoting a healthy metabolism.

In essence, while organic foods offer certain benefits, including potentially lower pesticide exposure and environmental advantages, they are not a magic bullet for weight loss. Successful weight management is best achieved through a balanced diet, portion control, and consistent exercise, rather than relying solely on the organic label of foods.

External links:

Tasting Table — 11 Myths About Organic Food, Debunked
https://www.tastingtable.com/952818/myths-about-organic-food-debunked/

proconguide — Organic Food Myths: Debunking Common Misconceptions
https://proconguide.com/organic-food-myths/

Better Health Channel — Weight loss - common myths
https://www.betterhealth.vic.gov.au/health/healthyliving/weight-loss-common-myths

The Healthy — Healthy Eating: 21 Food Myths You Still Think Are True
https://www.thehealthy.com/food/common-food-myths/

Organic — Organic Myths
https://organic.org/organic-myths/

Eating snacks is bad for weight loss

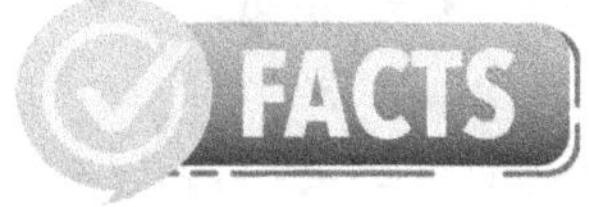

Healthy snacks can prevent overeating at meals and keep metabolism stable. It's the choice of snack that matters.

The idea that snacking is inherently bad for weight loss is a common misconception. In reality, healthy snacks can be a crucial part of a weight loss plan by preventing overeating during meals and keeping your metabolism stable.

Healthy snacks can help control hunger and prevent the urge to overeat at main meals. This is because snacking can keep your blood sugar levels steady, reducing the chances of extreme hunger, which often leads to overeating and poor food choices. For instance, incorporating snacks like an apple with peanut butter or Greek yogurt with berries provides a good balance of protein, fiber, and healthy fats that help keep you full longer.

Additionally, snacking can provide a steady stream of energy throughout the day, which is particularly beneficial if several hours pass between meals. This can prevent the dips in energy that might lead to consuming high-calorie, low-nutrient foods out of convenience.

The key is to choose snacks that are nutritious and in appropriate portions. Snacks high in protein and fiber, such as nuts, seeds, whole grains, fruits, and vegetables, are excellent choices. These snacks not only help maintain satiety but also provide essential nutrients that contribute to overall health. For example, pairing raw vegetables with hummus or having a handful of mixed nuts can be both satisfying and nourishing.

However, it's important to be mindful of the types and amounts of snacks consumed. Over-snacking or choosing high-calorie, low-nutrient snacks like chips or cookies can lead to weight gain and poor health outcomes. It's also beneficial to be aware of portion sizes and to avoid eating snacks directly from large packages to prevent overeating.

In summary, snacking can be a helpful tool for weight management when done thoughtfully. By choosing healthy, nutrient-dense snacks and being mindful of portions, snacking can support a balanced diet and prevent the pitfalls of extreme hunger and overeating at meals.

External links:

Mayo Clinic Connect — Snacking – Good, Bad, or Ugly for Weight Management?
https://connect.mayoclinic.org/blog/weight-management-1/newsfeed-post/snacking-good-bad-or-ugly-for-weight-management/

The Nutrition Source — The Science of Snacking
https://nutritionsource.hsph.harvard.edu/snacking/

Eat This Not That — 9 Ways Snacking Can Help You Lose Weight, Say Dietitians
https://www.eatthis.com/snacking-can-help-you-lose-weight/

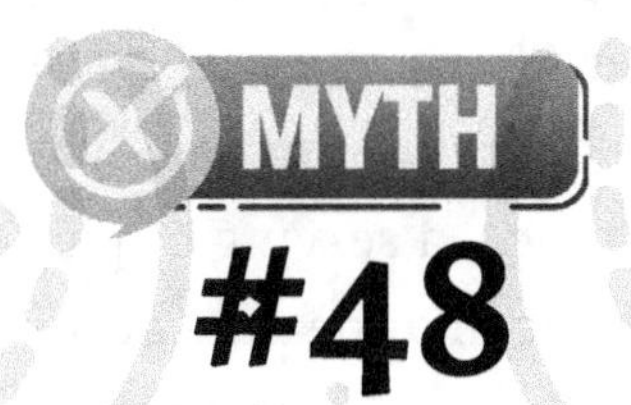

You need to avoid all your favorite foods permanently

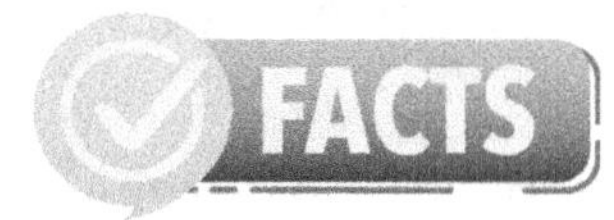

Moderation and portion control allow for occasional indulgences without sabotaging weight loss.

The belief that you need to avoid all your favorite foods permanently to achieve weight loss is a widespread myth. In reality, incorporating your favorite foods in moderation and practicing portion control can actually support long-term weight management and prevent feelings of deprivation that often lead to overeating.

One of the key strategies is to practice mindful eating. This involves paying full attention to the experience of eating and savoring each bite. For instance, enjoying a small piece of chocolate slowly can satisfy your craving without the need to consume large quantities. This approach helps you enjoy your favorite treats while maintaining control over your portions.

Moderation means including small amounts of your favorite foods within a balanced diet. This not only makes your diet more enjoyable but also more sustainable. Instead of completely cutting out foods like pizza, ice cream, or cookies, you can learn to incorporate them occasionally in a controlled manner. For example, having a scoop of ice cream once a week or a slice of pizza as part of a balanced meal can prevent feelings of deprivation and the subsequent binge eating that often follows strict dieting rules.

Portion control is another effective tool. Using smaller plates, measuring out servings, and being aware of actual portion sizes can help you manage your intake without eliminating the foods you love. For instance, a serving of pasta should fit within two cupped hands, and a serving of fat, like peanut butter, should be about the size of your thumb. By being mindful of these portions, you can enjoy a variety of foods while still adhering to your calorie goals.

The Mayo Clinic highlights that balance and moderation are essential. Instead of adopting a deprivation mindset, focus on filling up on nutritious foods like fruits and vegetables, and save your indulgent treats for when you truly crave them. This balanced approach can help you maintain a healthy diet and achieve your weight loss goals without feeling restricted.

External links:

Mayo Clinic Diet — Eat what you love and still lose weight
https://diet.mayoclinic.org/us/blog/2022/eat-what-you-love-and-still-lose-weight/

Medicine LibreTexts — 2.2: Myths and Misconceptions about Nutrition
https://med.libretexts.org/Bookshelves/Health_and_Fitness/Contemporary_Health_Issues_(Baker)/02%3A_Nutritional_Health/2.02%3A_Myths_and_Misconceptions_about_Nutrition

Nerd Fitness — How to Portion Control (for Weight Loss)
https://www.nerdfitness.com/blog/how-to-portion-control-how-to-lose-weight-with-portion-control/

Nia Shanks — Eating in Moderation: How to Do It Right
https://niashanks.com/eating-in-moderation/

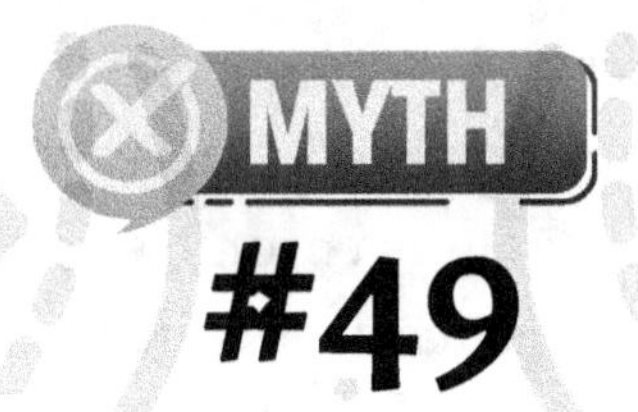

Dieting is the only way to lose weight

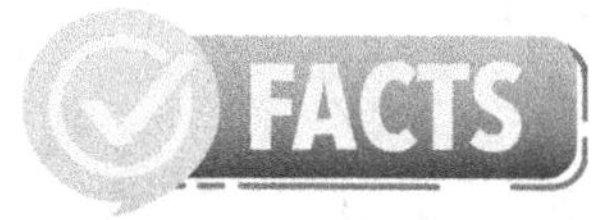

A combination of diet, exercise, sleep, and stress management is the most effective approach to weight loss.

The notion that dieting alone is the key to weight loss is a common misconception. In reality, a holistic approach that combines diet, exercise, sleep, and stress management is the most effective way to achieve and maintain weight loss.

While diet plays a crucial role in weight management, relying solely on calorie restriction can lead to temporary results and potential nutrient deficiencies. A balanced diet should include a variety of nutritious foods, such as vegetables, fruits, whole grains, lean proteins, and healthy fats. This not only supports weight loss but also ensures your body gets the necessary nutrients for overall health.

Regular physical activity is another critical component. Exercise helps burn calories, boosts metabolism, and preserves muscle mass, which is vital for long-term weight maintenance. Both aerobic exercises, like walking or cycling, and strength training are beneficial. Strength training, in particular, helps build muscle, which can increase your metabolic rate and support weight loss.

Sleep and stress management also significantly impact weight management. Poor sleep can disrupt hormones that regulate appetite, leading to increased hunger and cravings. Managing stress is equally important, as chronic stress can lead to emotional eating and weight gain. Techniques such as meditation, yoga, or simply ensuring you get adequate sleep can help manage these factors.

In conclusion, while dieting is an important aspect of weight loss, incorporating regular exercise, ensuring adequate sleep, and managing stress are equally crucial for achieving sustainable results. This comprehensive approach not only aids in weight loss but also promotes overall health and well-being.

External links:

WW — 10 Weight Loss Myths | Starvation Mode + More
https://www.weightwatchers.com/us/blog/weight-loss/top-weight-loss-myths

Mayo Clinic — Weight loss: 6 strategies for success
https://www.mayoclinic.org/healthy-lifestyle/weight-loss/in-depth/weight-loss/art-20047752

NIDDK — Eating & Physical Activity to Lose or Maintain Weight
https://www.niddk.nih.gov/health-information/weight-management/adult-overweight-obesity/eating-physical-activity

Mayo Clinic Diet — 5 ways to increase weight loss on Wegovy
https://diet.mayoclinic.org/us/blog/2024/5-ways-to-increase-weight-loss-on-wegovy/

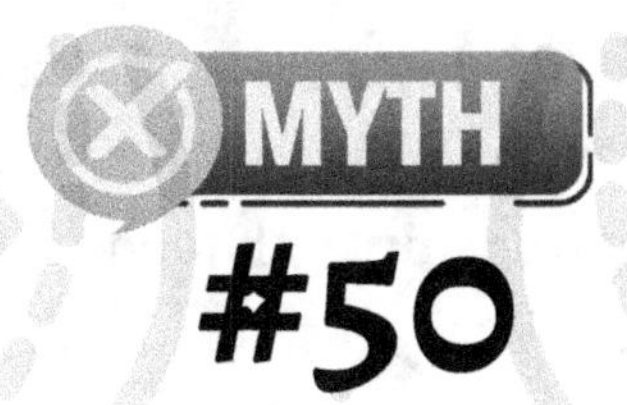

Rapid weight loss is always better

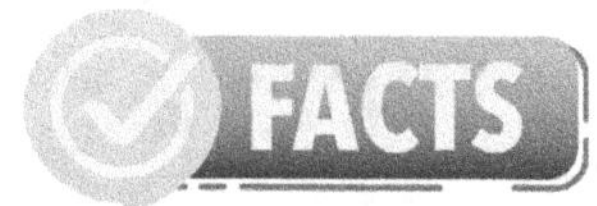

Slow and steady weight loss is more sustainable and healthier, reducing the risk of rebound weight gain and promoting lasting habits.

The belief that rapid weight loss is always better is a common myth. In reality, slow and steady weight loss is generally more sustainable and healthier. This approach reduces the risk of rebound weight gain and promotes the establishment of lasting healthy habits.

Rapid weight loss often involves extreme diets and intense exercise regimens, which can lead to a quick reduction in weight but are hard to maintain long-term. When people lose weight too quickly, they often regain it once they return to their normal eating patterns. This is partly because rapid weight loss can lead to muscle loss and a slower metabolism, making it easier to regain weight.

In contrast, slow and steady weight loss allows the body to adjust gradually to changes, promoting fat loss while preserving muscle mass. This method is more likely to lead to lasting weight management. A gradual approach, typically defined as losing 1-2 pounds per week, encourages the development of healthy eating and exercise habits that are sustainable over time.

Moreover, slower weight loss reduces the risk of negative side effects such as nutrient deficiencies, fatigue, and irritability, which are common with rapid weight loss. It also helps in maintaining a healthier relationship with food and reduces the psychological stress associated with drastic dietary restrictions.

Studies have shown that individuals who lose weight gradually are more likely to keep it off in the long run. This approach allows for the incorporation of balanced nutrition, regular physical activity, adequate sleep, and stress management, all of which contribute to overall health and well-being.

External links:

HMR Program — The Myth of Slow and Steady Weight Loss
https://www.hmrprogram.com/resources/staying-on-track/myth-of-slow-steady-weight-loss

WW — The Biggest Loser study: Why slow & steady weight loss wins the race
https://www.weightwatchers.com/us/blog/weight-loss/the-biggest-loser-study-why-slow-steady-weight-loss-wins-the-race

Home — Rapid vs. Slow Weight Loss: Which is better for Long-Term Progress?
https://phase-iv.com/rapid-vs-slow-weight-loss-which-is-better-for-long-term-progress/

Bibliography

Why We Get Fat: And What to Do About It by Gary Taubes

The Obesity Code: Unlocking the Secrets of Weight Loss by Dr. Jason Fung

Intuitive Eating: A Revolutionary Program that Works by Evelyn Tribole and Elyse Resch

The Diet Myth: Why the Secret to Health and Weight Loss is Already in Your Gut by Tim Spector

Good Calories, Bad Calories: Fats, Carbs, and the Controversial Science of Diet and Health by Gary Taubes

The Complete Guide to Fasting: Heal Your Body Through Intermittent, Alternate-Day, and Extended Fasting by Dr. Jason Fung and Jimmy Moore

The Case Against Sugar by Gary Taubes

Body Respect: What Conventional Health Books Get Wrong, Leave Out, and Just Plain Fail to Understand about Weight by Linda Bacon and Lucy Aphramor

Salt Sugar Fat: How the Food Giants Hooked Us by Michael Moss

Mindless Eating: Why We Eat More Than We Think by Brian Wansink

Fat Chance: Beating the Odds Against Sugar, Processed Food, Obesity, and Disease by Dr. Robert Lustig

The End of Dieting: How to Live for Life by Dr. Joel Fuhrman

The New Rules of Lifting for Women: Lift Like a Man, Look Like a Goddess by Lou Schuler, Cassandra Forsythe, and Alwyn Cosgrove

In Defense of Food: An Eater's Manifesto by Michael Pollan

The China Study: The Most Comprehensive Study of Nutrition Ever Conducted and the Startling Implications for Diet, Weight Loss, and Long-Term Health by T. Colin Campbell and Thomas M. Campbell II

The Blue Zones Solution: Eating and Living Like the World's Healthiest People by Dan Buettner

How Not to Die: Discover the Foods Scientifically Proven to Prevent and Reverse Disease by Dr. Michael Greger

Wheat Belly: Lose the Wheat, Lose the Weight, and Find Your Path Back to Health by Dr. William Davis

Grain Brain: The Surprising Truth about Wheat, Carbs, and Sugar – Your Brain's Silent Killers by Dr. David Perlmutter

Eat Fat, Get Thin: Why the Fat We Eat Is the Key to Sustained Weight Loss and Vibrant Health by Dr. Mark Hyman

Always Hungry?: Conquer Cravings, Retrain Your Fat Cells, and Lose Weight Permanently by Dr. David Ludwig

The Big Fat Surprise: Why Butter, Meat and Cheese Belong in a Healthy Diet by Nina Teicholz

The Plant Paradox: The Hidden Dangers in 'Healthy' Foods That Cause Disease and Weight Gain by Dr. Steven R. Gundry

The Four-Hour Body: An Uncommon Guide to Rapid Fat-Loss, Incredible Sex, and Becoming Superhuman by Timothy Ferriss

Clean: The Revolutionary Program to Restore the Body's Natural Ability to Heal Itself by Dr. Alejandro Junger

Eat to Live: The Amazing Nutrient-Rich Program for Fast and Sustained Weight Loss by Dr. Joel Fuhrman

Metabolical: The Lure and the Lies of Processed Food, Nutrition, and Modern Medicine by Dr. Robert Lustig

The Hungry Brain: Outsmarting the Instincts That Make Us Overeat by Stephan Guyenet

The Fast Metabolism Diet: Eat More Food and Lose More Weight by Haylie Pomroy

Rethinking Thin: The New Science of Weight Loss—and the Myths and Realities of Dieting by Gina Kolata

Why Diets Make Us Fat: The Unintended Consequences of Our Obsession with Weight Loss by Sandra Aamodt

Bright Line Eating: The Science of Living Happy, Thin & Free by Susan Peirce Thompson

Fat for Fuel: A Revolutionary Diet to Combat Cancer, Boost Brain Power, and Increase Your Energy by Dr. Joseph Mercola

The Complete Ketogenic Diet for Beginners: Your Essential Guide to Living the Keto Lifestyle by Amy Ramos

The Alkaline Reset Cleanse: The 7-Day Reboot for Unlimited Energy, Rapid Weight Loss, and the Prevention of Degenerative Disease by Ross Bridgeford

Eat Drink and Be Healthy: The Harvard Medical School Guide to Healthy Eating by Dr. Walter Willett

Referenced Sites

Throughout this book, we've cited numerous articles and resources to provide you with accurate and insightful information. Below is a list of the home pages for all the referenced sites, along with the myth numbers where their articles are mentioned. Visit these sites to explore further and access the wealth of knowledge they offer.

allnutritious.com
anytimefitness.com
askthescientists.com
atkins.com
barbend.com
beaumont.org
betterhealth.vic.gov.au
bistromd.com
blog.myfitnesspal.com
bmj.com
bodybuilding.com
bodybuilding-wizard.com
buoyhealth.com
chefsresource.com
connect.mayoclinic.org
curejoy.com
diet.mayoclinic.org
dietdoctor.com
dietitiankea.com
discover.texasrealfood.com
drbrahma.com
eatthis.com
elitefts.com
essentialsportsnutrition.com
everydayhealth.com
factmyth.com
foodbornewellness.com
fruitsandveggies.org

globalnews.ca

gotmilk.com

gwrymca.org

habs.uq.edu.au

health.clevelandclinic.org

healthwellbeing.com

henryford.com

hindustantimes.com

hmrprogram.com

home.myshapa.com

houstonmethodist.org

hsph.harvard.edu

hub.jhu.edu

indiatoday.in

iowaclinic.com

iowafarmbureau.com

joincalibrate.com

leanbodygoals.com

lifemd.com

livescience.com

livestrong.com

lorieeberwellnesscoaching.com

mayoclinic.org

mayoclinichealthsystem.org

mdanderson.org

mdlinx.com

med.libretexts.org

medicalxpress.com

medlineplus.gov

merakilane.com

michiganmedicine.org

mindbodygreen.com

my.vanderbilthealth.com

myauthentikspoon.com

nccih.nih.gov

nerdfitness.com

news.harvard.edu

newsnetwork.mayoclinic.org

nhs.uk

niashanks.com

niddk.nih.gov

nutritionfacts.org

nutritionist-resource.org.uk

nutritionletter.tufts.edu

nutritionsource.hsph.harvard.edu

organic.org

pbmchealth.org

pennmedicine.org

phase-iv.com

phhp.ufl.edu

piedmont.org

precisionnutrition.com

preventivemedicinedaily.com

proconguide.com

qilo.co

sciencedaily.com

shapescale.com

simple.life

simplegreensmoothies.com

sites.miamioh.edu

sportsmedicineweekly.com

stack.com

strengthzonetraining.com

sydney.edu.au

tastingtable.com

thebalancednutritionist.com

thehealthy.com

todaysdietitian.com

uab.edu

uchicagomedicine.org

verywellfit.com

weightmatters.ie
weightwatchers.com
well-choices.com
yalescientific.org
zozofit.com

About the series

The *"50 Myths About..."* series debunks common misconceptions across a wide range of topics. Each book in the series provides evidence-based insights, challenging popular myths and offering readers a fresh perspective. Whether exploring architecture, science, history, or other fields, these books aim to educate, engage, and inspire curiosity. Perfect for anyone eager to uncover the truth and deepen their understanding, the *"50 Myths About..."* series is your go-to guide for myth-busting knowledge.

Already published:

- *50 Myths About Architecture and Buildings:* Unveiling the Truth Behind Common Architectural Misconceptions